POLICY STUDIES IN EMPLOYMENT AND WELFARE NUMBER 27

General Editor: Sar A. Levitan

ENTRY-LEVEL HEALTH OCCUPATIONS: DEVELOPMENT AND FUTURE

Harold M. Goldstein and
Morris A. Horowitz

The Johns Hopkins University Press, Baltimore and London

To Lila and Jean

Manufactured in the United States of America

The Johns Hopkins University Press, Baltimore, Maryland 21218
The Johns Hopkins Press Ltd., London

Library of Congress Catalog Card Number 76–41270
ISBN 0-8018-1911-3 (hardcover)
ISBN 0-8018-1912-1

Library of Congress Cataloging in Publication data will be found on the last printed page of this book.

This study was prepared under a grant from the Ford Foundation

Contents

Tables

Figure

Acknowledgments

A significant portion of the information presented in this report has been acquired by the authors over the past ten years in their work in the Department of Economics, and more recently in the Center for Medical Manpower Studies, both at Northeastern University, Boston. Continued support for studies of health manpower has come from the Office of Research and Development, Employment and Training Administration (formerly the Manpower Administration), U.S. Department of Labor, and for this we are indebted to Dr. Howard Rosen and Mr. William Throckmorton of that office. We also wish to express our appreciation to Professor Sar A. Levitan of the Center for Social Policy Studies, the George Washington University, for his encouragement in this project.

We wish to express our appreciation for the collection, analysis, and supply of international health data to Elio Guzzanti, M.D., Superintendent, the United Hospitals of Rome, Audace Gemelli, Professor and Editor of *I Problemi della Sicurezza Sociale,* and Enzo Lancia, M.D., of the United Hospitals of Rome.

We are indebted to a number of persons for their efforts in the preparation of this manuscript. They are Kathleen A. Calore, Patricia McCarville and Alec Cheloff of the Center for Medical Manpower Studies, William A. Frolich and Margaret Courtney of the Northeastern University Press, Diane Ullius Jarrett, Henry K. Tom and James S. Johnston of the Johns Hopkins University Press.

This study does not necessarily represent the official opinion or policy of the Employment and Training Administration or Northeastern University. The authors are solely responsible for the contents of the study.

ENTRY-LEVEL
HEALTH OCCUPATIONS:
DEVELOPMENT AND FUTURE

1

Introduction

Unemployment in the United States is endemic to various ethnic minorities, generally those classified as disadvantaged. Although there are substantial numbers of employed poor, poverty for many others is the result of unemployment — the inability to locate and hold a meaningful job. Such unemployment exists in the best of times. And with unemployment widespread throughout the nation, the ethnic minorities, especially the blacks, have been particularly hard hit.

Although poverty is nationwide, the incidence of poverty is related to age, color, sex of family head, work status, and educational attainment. Blacks are three times as likely as whites to be poor; families headed by women are nearly five times as likely to be poor as families headed by men; and when the head of the family has eight years of schooling or less, the incidence of poverty is four times greater than in families headed by a person with some college education.[1] The general relationship between poverty and unemployment is commonly accepted. Although there have been many government efforts and programs attacking the problems of poverty, poverty is still with us, and so also are the unemployment problems of the poor and the disadvantaged.

Meaningful, high-paying jobs with opportunities for advancement do not seem to be readily available for the black, or the woman, or

1

the teenager, or the high school dropout; and these are often the characteristics of the poor and the disadvantaged. Can our society attain the heights of scientific success yet not be able to develop meaningful job opportunities for its disadvantaged?

Even with high unemployment rates jobs are generally available in the central cities, where substantial portions of the unemployed minorities live. These are the jobs of the secondary labor market, characterized by low pay, menial tasks, and no possibility of job advancement. Such jobs would include the dishwasher, the gas station attendant, the sweeper in a retail establishment. Because of the nature of these jobs there is high labor turnover, for even the employed poor find it difficult to stay with such jobs for any length of time.

What our economy must provide are expanding industries capable of employing large numbers of these minorities, even those with such handicaps as the lack of a high school diploma. We feel that the health care industry is such an industry. We intend to show in this study that the health care industry is expanding, despite the unemployment crunch in most other sectors of the economy. And because of the likely adoption of a national health insurance program, the industry is likely to expand even more rapidly in the future. We also intend to show that the industry has large numbers of meaningful jobs and occupations that currently exclude ethnic minorities and other disadvantaged but that many of these persons could fill satisfactorily.

The evidence is not uniform across the nation. For various reasons employment barriers have been erected by hospital administrators and by occupational groups. Education requirements, training and experience requirements, and certification and licensing requirements are common methods of excluding or limiting part of the potential supply of workers. And the disadvantaged are usually the first to be excluded. Are these hiring requirements valid in terms of the functions to be performed? In many cases validity would be difficult to prove because the end product, the health of the patient, is difficult to measure and is always dependent on the work of various groups. However, there are significant examples of hospitals where education and training requirements have been lowered without any effect on patient care. If the hiring requirements can be lowered in some hospitals, one can legitimately assume that they can also be lowered in many or all other hospitals. Eliminating the high school diploma as a hiring-in requirement for entry-level occupations will open a substantial number of jobs to the disadvantaged.

As the occupational structure of the industry now stands, there are not very many opportunities for upward mobility or even lateral mobility. Entry-level jobs generally end up as dead-end jobs. Recently, however, experiments have been made in restructuring the occupational hierarchy of hospitals and in creating meaningful occupational ladders. In our judgment the experiments have been relatively successful. But widespread changes across the nation will require time and considerable effort and pressure by the government and by society. It can be done, and it must be done. Meaningful job opportunities can be made available in the health care industry for the disadvantaged without any decrease in standards of patient care.

Definition of Scope

As in many industries of our market economy, personnel in the health care industry ranges from the unskilled to the professional and administrator. However, unlike most industries, there is no general agreement in the health industry as to who are the professionals and who come under other broad classifications. Fifty years ago it seemed clear that physicians (and probably dentists and pharmacists) were the only professionals of the industry. With the growth and changes of the past thirty years, there is considerable uncertainty as to what classifications other than physicians are to be considered professionals, and what distinctions if any should be made among the numerous classifications that are not considered professional.

To some the term *professional* is restricted to the physician alone, since it is the only occupation in the industry that requires a college education plus post-graduate medical school training. This would nicely fit the dictionary definition of the learned professions as being theology, law, and medicine. In order to classify the other occupations in the industry, such terms as *paraprofessional, subprofessional, semiprofessional, paramedical,* and *auxiliary* have been developed. But because there is no consistent pattern of usage, these terms have caused confusion and sometimes bitterness among various occupational groups in the industry. By some definitions the term *paraprofessional* (or paramedical) includes registered nurses, sanitary engineers, radiologic technologists and technicians, and even veterinarians and dentists. The terms *auxiliary* and *ancillary* have been used by some to describe a broad category of workers who are considered to be distinctly subordinate to those in the professional and paramedical categories. The term *subprofessional* has probably caused the most problems because of the connotation of the word. It tends to diminish the status of the groups it encompasses and may inhibit the development of a sense of responsibility in the employees of occupations so classified.

Many health occupational groups have organized themselves into unions and professional associations, and they consider themselves to be professional, although they could hardly meet the time-honored definition of theology, law, and medicine. Certainly many so-called professional groups function in the United States as highly structured organizations that have key interests in certification and accreditation requirements, although in numerous instances their members would not meet the criteria of graduate education, undergraduate education or, in some instances, even a high school diploma.

By sheer numbers the registered nurse (RN) now plays an important role among health providers, but there is no agreement whether the nurse is a professional. In some instances she or he might have a master's degree or, in a larger number of cases, a bachelor of science degree. In most instances, however, the RN is a graduate of a three-year program; even two-year programs are still quite common. Is the principal criterion for classification a license or certification that specifies a minimum level of education? Or are the duties and functions performed the key to the classification? Again, there is no agreed-upon answer. However, at this point it should be noted that there is a tremendous overlap in the performance of medical functions among all levels of health personnel, from the physician to the registered nurse to the entry-level health employee; and almost all are likely to consider themselves professional.

An example of the problem is the electrocardiographic (EKG) or electroencephalographic (EEG) technician who performs a full range of medical functions. In numerous instances persons in this classification have no more than secondary-school educations (and in some cases even less) but have been trained on the job in the hospital by a cardiologist. After some years of experience in such a position, the EKG or EEG technicians are likely to consider themselves professionals. By what standards does one classify these technicians positions as subprofessional or paraprofessional?

During and immediately after World War II it was common to classify most health care occupations, save the physician, as paramedical personnel. This term included all health-related occupations from the registered nurse down to the entry-level medical or surgical nursing aides. During the late 1960's the term fell into disrepute, principally because members of many occupations subsumed by the term believed it downgraded their image and prestige. The word *paramedical* was dropped, and in its stead was adopted the phrase *allied health*. The striving for status and recognition by various occupations soon called this phrase into question: there was a desire to be independent and not allied to any specific subgroup or occupation. By 1975 there was a growing move to adopt the term *health care personnel* to cover all occupations related to health, including that of physician.

In view of these changes this report will use the terms *allied health* or *health* personnel or occupations. These terms will include all those persons in the industry who directly relate to the patient — "laying-hands-on." Such a title would cover the whole range of health workers from the physician extender (such as the pediatric nurse practitioner and the graduate registered nurse who had four or five years of formal schooling after secondary school) to the entry-level nurse's aide or assistant and the laboratory assistant (who may have as little as a high school education plus on-the-job training and/ or in-service education). In a number of notable instances even the high school education is not an absolute requirement for entry-level positions among health care providers.

In 1910 there were essentially only three members of the health care team — physicians, nurses, and aides. By 1974 the figure had risen to well over 450 individual health care occupations,[2] and the most current estimate puts the figure at 600.[3] However, it is very likely that many health occupations have duplicate titles and are therefore listed more than once. Nevertheless, with such a range of job titles it is difficult to rank them accurately as to which are professional and which are entry-level positions.

There are a number of factors by which one can classify who is and who is not a professional. The following are some criteria:

1. Formal education and examination is required.

2. Certification or licensing is required.

3. Regional or national associations have been established.

4. There is a code of professional performance and ethics.

5. There is a body of systematic scientific knowledge and/or technical skill.

6. Individuals within the category can function with some degree of autonomy, under the assumption that they have the expertise to make decisions in their area of competence.

By one or more of these factors most of the health care occupations could be classified as professional.

Although the focus of this study is principally on the entry-level classifications, there is no unanimous agreement as to which classifications may be considered ports of entry for the unskilled and untrained. In some hospitals in some geographic areas certain occupations are considered entry-level, and with training the employees are moved up an occupational ladder. But there is no uniform pattern of hiring-in or of moving up a ladder. The occupation of surgical technician may be cited as an example. In most instances the surgical technician was first employed by the health provider in an entry-level occupation, such as nurse's aide. She or he could have functioned as a nurse's aide for several months or a year before being assigned to the surgery department. It is not unusual for persons in entry-level jobs to be exposed to on-the-job training or in-service education programs in the department of surgery, where the training is provided by staff surgeons. At some point in the training the person may be classified as a surgical technician. This situation is usual in the United States Navy, where after two or three years of on-the-job training an entry-level aide finds himself a functioning member of a surgical team. There is no uniform pattern in the industry of hiring-in, of training, or of promotion. The extent to which opportunities exist and the ways to expand these opportunities are what this study is all about.

Setting the Scene — the Industry

From the point of view of most social scientists, the purchase of health care is not much different from the purchase of other goods or services. In a market economy, such as prevails in the United States, demand — the willingness and ability to purchase goods and services — depends on taste, price, income, and the availability of substitutes. The health care industry differs from other industries in that the purchase of health services is highly inelastic. At some income levels and above, the demand for health care services is probably highly inelastic, whereas at the lower income levels there is some elasticity. Low-income families may forego health checkups and necessary medical care when the price is high. However, in emergencies — such as a ruptured appendix or a broken leg — the demand for medical service is there, regardless of price. And in such situations there is little opportunity to shop for the best "buy." The only substitute for health care is neglect, and relatively few persons are prepared to select this alternative when a matter is judged to be serious. Another interesting and relatively unusual aspect of the market for health services is that demand for services is often determined by the supplier of the service. When a physician informs a patient that additional visits are necessary or that an operation is needed, a demand for additional health services is created.

The health care industry is further complicated by numerous other social implications. For many persons the use of health care facilities and services is based on a nonrational decision that is made with little if any knowledge of the marketplace. In the early 1900's the physician was quite likely to be one of the relatively small number of educated persons in the community, and his judgment was rarely questioned. It was assumed that he had the solutions to all health problems. Over the last decade many American consumers of health care have raised considerable doubts about the near deification of physicians. However, the health care expectations of consumers remain unrealistically high. Americans have been led to believe that physicians, hospitals, and health care services know the answers to all medical problems and have a very positive impact on health. Needless to say, such is not necessarily the case. Most people who consider themselves ill do recover regardless of whether they are exposed to physicians, hospitals, or any other part of the health care system. A certain number of those individuals who consider themselves ill are terminal cases for whom exposure to the health care system will be of no benefit. Only in a percentage of cases can the health care service be of a positive nature. Most physicians have been aware of this situation for a number of years, yet there have been no serious attempts to dispel the aura that surrounds the physician and the hospital.

Society appears to place a high priority on health care service, yet the best of care is not always available to the poor and to various ethnic and disadvantaged groups. Health is often spoken of as the most important goal of society, yet we do relatively little to improve the delivery system so that health resources are distributed equitably. In the allocation of government expenditures it readily becomes clear that the health of the nation does not have a very high priority. And with the available information about the effects of smoking and drinking on health, it is also clear that many people do not give health a top priority.[4]

Physicians are without doubt the captains of the health care team, and there is no question that the whole industry hinges on them. The physician is the representative model consistently emulated by all other groups in the health care industry. Therefore, any discussion of allied health personnel must begin with some recognition and understanding of this leadership role.

Until the nineteenth century hospitals in the United States functioned primarily for the poor, the aged, and the mentally ill. The well-to-do took care of their ill at home. The status of all hospital personnel, including entry-level groups, was governed in great measure by the philanthropic nature of the hospitals. Few if any restrictions were placed on the growing number of hospitals established between the seventeenth century and the first half of the twentieth century. In fact, until the 1960's hospital construction had the enthusiastic support of all levels of government, health providers, and the consuming public. As a result the number of hospitals, beds, allied health personnel, and physicians grew haphazardly during this period to meet what apparently was seen as the American consumers' infinite capacity to utilize available services and facilities. How much value all this had in terms of health is moot. Of the estimated 3,500 physicians in the United States in 1775, only 400 held medical degrees.[5]

In the late nineteenth century American hospitals and physicians locked horns over the issue of hospital outpatient departments for the poor. At this time well over 95 percent of the physicians were in private practice, and they viewed the competition from outpatient clinics as a threat to their practice and income. The physicians won the battle, and as a result the development of outpatient departments and ambulatory facilities was neglected until the mid-1940's.

It was only after the publication of *The Flexner Report*[6] in 1910 that serious attention was directed toward the regulation of medical schools and other schools of allied health manpower and toward the general improvement of standards in hospitals. Between 1910 and 1930, as a direct result of the recommendations of *The Flexner Report*, the number of medical schools was reduced from 148 to 76, based on the criterion that they had to provide reasonably satisfactory medical education.

The Flexner Report resulted not only in an improved education for physicians and traditional allied health personnel, but also in a relative decrease in the number of physicians. These changes, along with the economic prosperity that came after World War I, resulted in a lessening of competition between physicians and hospitals. From that time on, the increased utilization of sophisticated medical innovation and technology ensured the growing reliance of the physician on a well-equipped and staffed hospital. In this period the merits of having a staff of full-time physicians (contractual physicians) in a hospital became more obvious, and by 1974 over twenty-five percent of the practicing physicians in the United States were contractual physicians.

Since the end of World War II there has been an enormous increase in third-party medical coverage. This fact, in addition to the quickening pace of technological development in medicine, provided the basis for a vast expansion of hospital services and a moderate increase in bed capacity in the United States. An indication of the magnitude of growth in hospitals and their utilization is shown in Table I. The number of hospital beds and the average daily census of hospital patients peaked in the mid-1960's and has shown rather steady but moderate declines since that time. Both of these measures, computed per 1,000 population, have shown a steady decline since 1946. The annual number of hospital admissions, in absolute figures and per 1,000 population, showed a steady rise over the whole period from 1945 to 1973.

Over the five-year period from 1968 through 1973 there has been a leveling off of hospital construction and bed capacity. Not only was there an overall reduction of 7.7 percent in the number of beds, but the average daily census declined by 13.7 percent, and the occupancy rate dropped by 6.5 percent as well. The number of admissions, however, rose by 15.4 percent, and the number of outpatient visits increased by 49.6 percent (see Table 2).

The overall decrease in the number of active staffed beds took place in noncommunity hospitals, which experienced a 5.1 percent decrease. Community hospitals showed an increase of 2.2 percent; community hospitals are defined as all nonfederal, short-term general hospitals whose facilities are available to the public. The 5.1 percent decrease in noncommunity beds came about primarily in psychiatric (7.7 percent) and tuberculosis (23.1 percent) hospitals.[7]

The growth trends in American hospitals with respect to personnel and finances over the last three decades have been significant. The number of hospital personnel, principally allied health personnel, increased from 830,000 in 1946 to 1,840,000 in 1963 and to 2,769,000 in 1973. Total hospital payrolls rose from $1.103 billion in 1946 to $7.270 billion in 1963 and $21.330 billion in 1973.[8]

One of the more significant shifts that occurred during the postwar period was the substantial increase in hospital-based outpatient utilization. In 1963 the number of outpatient visits totaled 118,238,000; by 1973 it was 233,555,000, an increase of 97.5 percent. It is estimated that over 80 percent of this shift was due to

Table 1. Utilization Trends in All United States Hospitals for Selected Years, 1946-1973

Year	Hospital Beds		Average Daily Census		Admissions	
	Number	per 1,000 Population	Number	per 1,000 Population	Number	per 1,000 Population
1946	1,436,000	10.2	1,142,000	8.0	15,675,000	110.4
1950	1,456,000	9.6	1,253,000	8.2	18,483,000	121.4
1955	1,604,000	9.6	1,363,000	8.2	21,073,000	127.0
1960	1,658,000	9.1	1,402,000	7.7	25,027,000	138.5
1961	1,670,000	9.1	1,393,000	7.6	25,474,000	138.7
1962	1,689,000	9.0	1,407,000	7.5	26,531,000	142.2
1963	1,702,000	9.0	1,430,000	7.5	27,502,000	145.3
1964	1,696,000	8.8	1,421,000	7.4	28,266,000	147.3
1965	1,704,000	8.7	1,403,000	7.2	28,812,000	148.3
1966	1,679,000	8.5	1,398,000	7.1	29,151,000	148.3
1967	1,671,000	8.4	1,380,000	6.9	29,361,000	147.7
1968	1,663,000	8.2	1,378,000	6.8	29,766,000	148.3
1969	1,650,000	8.1	1,346,000	6.6	30,729,000	151.6
1970	1,616,000	7.8	1,298,000	6.3	31,759,000	155.0
1971	1,556,000	7.5	1,237,000	5.9	32,664,000	157.7
1972	1,550,000	7.4	1,209,000	5.8	33,265,000	159.2
1973	1,535,000	7.3	1,189,000	5.6	34,352,000	163.3

Source: Calculated from American Hospital Association *Hospital Statistics*, Annual Survey, 1974 Edition (Chicago: AHA, 1974), pp. 19-21. Population estimates used to calculate above figures from U.S. Department of Commerce, Bureau of the Census, *Statistical Abstract of the United States, 1974*. (Washington: Government Printing Office, 1974), p. 5.

Table 2. Selected Measures of Hospital Facilities and Utilization in
United States, 1968, 1971, and 1973

	Year			Percent Change		
	1968	1971	1973	1968-1971	1971-1973	1968-1973
Number of hospitals	7,138.0	7,097.0	7,123.0	−0.6	0.4	−0.2
Beds (in thousands)	1,663.0	1,556.0	1,535.0	−6.4	−1.3	−7.7
Average number of beds per hospital	233.0	219.0	215.5	−6.0	−1.6	−7.5
Admissions (in thousands)	29,766.0	32,664.0	34,352.0	9.7	5.2	15.4
Average daily census (in thousands)	1,378.0	1,237.0	1,189.0	−10.2	−3.9	−13.7
Occupancy percentage	82.9	79.5	77.5	−4.1	−2.5	−6.5
Outpatient visits (in thousands)	156,139.0[a]	199,725.0	233,555.0	27.9	16.9	49.6

Source: AHA, *Hospital Statistics,* 1974, pp. 19-21.

[a] Based on hospitals reporting outpatient visits.

the increased utilization of the ambulatory facilities of nonfederal short-term general and other special hospitals.

As noted above, during the 1970's there has been a reduced rate of growth in both hospitals and total bed capacity, due largely to the substantial increases in the cost of medical care. Some of the reasons for runaway health costs, especially hospital costs, are more obvious than others. Wage increases, the expansion of medical insurance programs, the relative maldistribution of physicians and allied health manpower, the implementation of new and more expensive medical techniques, and the relatively high profits of drug firms all have played a part in the spectacular price increases for medical care.

Because of the philanthropic origins of hospitals, some categories of health personnel still receive relatively low wages in comparison to their counterparts in the industrial sector. However, in general the earnings of health personnel have improved substantially in recent years, a fact that has caused significant increases in hospital costs. Skilled, semiskilled, and entry-level personnel — including such occupations as registered nurses (RNs), licensed practical nurses (LPNs), nurse's aides (NAs), technicians, and technologists — are the bulk of labor inputs, and their wages constitute the largest portion of total hospital costs. Hospitals are a very labor-intensive industry; that is, the lion's share of inputs and costs represents services performed by labor, although there has been an upward trend in the introduction of highly sophisticated and very expensive equipment. Costs of employing allied health personnel have increased significantly over the last decade, partly because of the unionization of these groups, especially in municipal hospitals. In addition, many groups of allied health workers have formed strong lobbying professional associations, which have used their leverage to increase salaries. Physician costs have increased more rapidly than the Consumer Price Index over the last decade in the United States, due largely to the fact that the supply of practicing physicians has not kept pace with the burgeoning demand for medical services.

Well over 75 percent of all hospital bills in the United States are covered by direct third-party payers (i.e., by medical insurance plans), and demand-pull inflation for medical care originates with such plans. The number of Americans covered by medical plans has increased substantially over the last twenty years, thereby increasing the demand for medical services, especially the services of the physician. More people believe they can now afford medical treatment, and they demand medical services.

Over the last decade there has been no increase in the number of physicians relative to the population, and the increased demand for medical services has tended to pull prices up. Hospital-related costs have simply been passed on to third-party payers, who in turn pass them on to the consumers. Only during the past five years has there been any concerted effort by the third-party payers to contain hospital costs.

By 1975 twenty-three of the fifty states had passed legislation establishing certificate of need (CON) committees, whose primary responsibility is to evaluate the genuine need for new hospitals and additions to existing hospitals. During the past several years these CON committees have had the effect of slowing the pace in the growth of hospital facilities and bed capacity. The approval of the CON committees is required if any public (federal, state, or local) funds are to be used in the medical facility. Despite the fact that significant political and private pressures are placed on the CON committees, they have had some success in slowing the expansion rate.

The experience of the Commonwealth of Massachusetts with its CON committee may indicate the effectiveness of such committees. The Massachusetts law was passed in 1972 and required that construction of health facilities costing more than $100,000 be approved by the CON committee. The law was established in response to a belief that too much of the funding available for health care was being spent on duplicative facilities in hospitals, diverting money that might be better used for outpatient care, home care services, and the like. In addition, a study completed in Massachusetts at about that time concluded that increasing the supply of beds generates its own subsquent demand to fill them.

A review of Massachusetts CON committee decisions conducted by the Massachusetts Department of Public Health found that in the first eighteen months under the new law:

1. The overall number of beds in general hospitals seeking certificates of need dropped by one-half of one percent, from 5,272 to 5,247. These hospitals had asked to increase their supply of beds by 9 percent to 5,715.

2. The CON committee approved increases in the numbers of general hospital beds devoted to psychiatric care, rehabilitation and extended care, diabetes, and alcoholism, though smaller than the increases proposed by the applicant hospitals.

3. Within the subcategory of acute-care hospital beds, hospitals applying for certificates of need had proposed a slight increase in the number of medical-surgical beds above the existing 4,053. The committee approved only 3,881 such beds, a reduction of 4 percent.[9]

The mere fact that a state requires a certificate of need appears to dampen the requests of hospitals for unnecessary expansion. It is to be hoped that, as these CON committees become more conversant with their responsibilities and powers, fewer unneeded hospitals, beds, or other medical facilities will be constructed.

One of the principal reasons that hospitals and medical care have recently received increased attention becomes apparent when one views the dollar value of activity in this field. Table 3 shows hospital expenditures as a percentage of gross national product (GNP) over the 1963-1973 period; this percentage rose from 1.86 in 1963 to 2.82 percent in 1973. Hospital expenditures in 1973 were $36.3 billion, which was an 11.1 percent increase over the 1972 figure. 1973 was the first year (with the exception of 1965) since 1963 that the rate of increase in the GNP exceeded the rate of increase in hospital expenditures. As mentioned above, this slow-down in hospital expenditures may in part be due to the increased attention devoted to this sector by certificate of need committees and third-party payers.

Table 3.   Hospital Expenditures as a Percentage of Gross National Product, 1963-1973

Year	GNP Amount (in billions)	GNP Percent Increase from Previous Year	Hospital Expenditures Amount (in millions)	Hospital Expenditures Percent Increase from Previous Year	Percentage of GNP
1963	$ 590.5	5.39	$10,956	8.17	1.86
1964	632.4	7.10	12,031	9.81	1.90
1965	684.9	8.30	12,948	7.62	1.89
1966	749.9	9.49	14,198	9.65	1.89
1967	793.9	5.87	16,395	15.47	2.07
1968	864.2	8.86	19,061	16.26	2.07
1969	930.3	7.65	22,103	15.96	2.38
1970	977.1	5.03	25,556	15.62	2.62
1971	1,055.5	8.02	28,812	12.74	2.73
1972	1,155.2	9.45	32,667	13.38	2.83
1973	1,289.1	11.59	36,290	11.09	2.82

Source: AHA *Hospital Statistics,* 1974, p. 6.

2

General Characteristics of Allied Health Personnel

In 1967 a detailed study of health personnel in the Greater Boston area by Professor Dean S. Ammer reached the following conclusions:[1]

1. Demand for allied health skills will outstrip supply in the foreseeable future.

2. Institutions deal with shortages by relying on part-time or less skilled help and by providing inferior services.

3. Shortages are not uniformly distributed.

4. Wider pay differentials should be encouraged.

5. Status-hungry allied health organizations indirectly contribute to the shortages.

6. Allied health middle management is poorly trained in techniques of administration.

Dr. Eli Ginzberg of Columbia University has some pointed comments to make about the health manpower situation. He notes that in virtually all fields dependent on trained manpower there are complaints of shortages, but that all will fail to meet their needs if they insist on perpetuating their old cumbersome patterns of staffing. Every field, including health care, finds the shifting of goals and redirection of resources difficult because of inflexibility, conservative attitudes, and weak leadership. He goes on to note that in a dynamic society time produces changes, and the institutions that were brought into being at an earlier period to cope with particular problems have in fact been eroded by alterations in the environment and in the priority needs of the population. To cope with these problems Ginzberg suggests such adjustments as eliminating or merging some tasks, reassigning tasks to personnel with less formal training and skills, substituting money for manpower in the performance of some functions, and transferring functions from the provider to the consumer of the service.[2]

In the same vein the Committee for Economic Development published a report in April 1973 entitled, *Building a National Health Care System,* which states:

Poor distribution, together with inadequate utilization, training, and organization, have aggravated the shortages of manpower in some areas while causing surpluses in others. Beyond some crude and increasingly doubtful ratios of professions to population, it is not even known how many people are now needed let alone how many would be needed under a better-organized system.[3]

If the market for health manpower operated efficiently with no artificial barriers, supply and demand would ultimately correct shortages. Institutions would act to retain or attract employees, restructure hiring standards and pay scales, institute training programs, and explore new sources of recruitment. However, in the real world this has not happened. Hospitals have not moved adequately to correct high turnover rates, job dissatisfaction, relatively low wage levels, and limited upward mobility. In general, shortages have tended to reflect budgeted positions and experience in hiring and turnover rather than the need for qualified health workers.

While the manpower shortages in the health care industry may be somewhat contrived, we must conclude that they do exist and will continue through the 1970's. We base this conclusion on the following facts:

1. Wage rates for health personnel, though still below those for manufacturing employees, have increased over the last five years at a rate higher than the average for all workers.[4]

2. Because of the nature of the service and the round-the-clock quality of the health industry, the normal attrition of the labor force

is very high, and for some occupations training is barely keeping pace with the need for replacements.

3. The enormous growth of technical knowledge has fragmented the occupations of health workers. At the beginning of this century the physician, the nurse, and the aide were probably the only recognized categories of health workers. In 1974 no less than 450 specialty groups, other than physicians, were to be found in the health care field. Despite the fact that inpatient occupancy rates are relatively constant, the number of health workers employed has increased substantially.

Excluding the physician, a substantial majority of the 4 million workers in the health manpower labor force are employed in hospitals, and a rather small minority employed in nursing and rest homes or in private laboratories. It was estimated in 1973 that over half of the health care employees were in low-income jobs paying about $4,000 a year, and that about 90 percent were women and 20 percent were black.

Relatively low wages and poor working conditions in the health care industry have resulted in a predominantly female work force. Two other characteristics of the industry helped account for the predominance of women in its work force, according to one study.[5] The research found a collection of small, quasi-independent labor markets for allied health manpower, composed of separate and rigidly defined occupations. At the lower skill levels, these markets tended to be local or regional, a factor that led to improper use of the less-skilled workers in dead-end jobs, with high turnover rates and job dissatisfaction. Moreover, the small employing units — predominantly charitable and nonprofit hospitals — generally had no administrative hierarchy separate from the professional hierarchy, and this condition further limited upward mobility and inhibited male employment. Thus, while the entry of more men into these occupations would undoubtedly tend to stabilize the work force and raise wages,[6] few men are attracted by jobs that offer low wages and little prospect of advancement.

High turnover and poor prospects of upward mobility were further documented in a 1968 study of health manpower.[7] Workers were asked what occupational level they hoped to attain and how long they had been working at their current occupations. Only in six of the eighteen jobs studied did a majority of workers expect to advance beyond their present job. And in thirteen of the jobs, at least two-fifths of the workers had been in the occupation for less than three years.[8] These findings suggest that there is high turnover in many allied health occupations and that many are, in fact, dead-end.

Occupational aspirations were probed further in a follow-up study.[9] In that study workers were asked whether they had a desire to rise to a higher level position and whether they believed they would attain this desire. Only licensed practical nurses, X-ray technicians, and laboratory technicians had any optimism about their prospects. Nearly all of the nurse's aides considered the job dead-end, even though more than three-fifths wished to advance. Only one-third were satisfied with the level of their job. One-fourth of the orderlies viewed the job as dead-end but wished to advance, whereas over three-fifths were satisfied. It should not be assumed, however, that everyone had a burning desire to climb some real or mythical occupational ladder. Many persons interviewed had become conditioned to their occupational status and were aware of the realistic limits to any upward mobility. Many entry-level health employees specifically stated that their job gave them no satisfaction but was simply a means toward their principal interest of earning a living. There is no doubt that over time the dead-end nature of their jobs conditioned their attitude.

This view suggests that attempts to establish career ladders will not succeed without concurrent efforts to provide motivation, education, and training, as well as appropriate salary scales. Since the present system has fostered limited expectations for career advancement, it is ultimately the responsibility of policy makers within the system to offer alternate career options to their personnel.

The basic elements or characteristics of entry-level health personnel would include —
1. high turnover
2. lack of opportunities for advancement
3. chronic employee shortages
4. functioning in an environment with a high degree of overlapping medical functions.

3

Utilization of Health Personnel

There are a number of crosscurrents in the health care industry that make it difficult to determine what is happening to the demand for allied health manpower and what will happen in the next few years. It is generally assumed, with little basis in fact, that the industry is expanding and that the demand for health care personnel will continue to grow. However, there are indications that hospitals in various parts of the nation are being underutilized. Hospital occupancy rates have declined over the past few years, and units of hospitals are being closed in various parts of the country. Yet there seems to be a marked increase in the use of the outpatient facilities of hospitals. In addition, there had been a growth of non-hospital-based health facilities, such as neighborhood health centers, health maintenance organizations, and extended care facilities, which employ growing numbers of health care personnel.

Changing Pattern of Employment

In an effort to determine the changing pattern of employment in the health industry as a guide to future planning, a study was undertaken in 1974 with the Boston area as the focus.[1] The principal objectives of this research project were (1) to determine what has happened during the five-year period 1968-1973 to the demand for manpower in selected occupational groups, as measured by employment in the cities of Boston and Cambridge; (2) to determine whether there is hospital overcapacity and, if so, what effects it has had on the employment and utilization of health manpower; and (3) to determine the effects on health manpower of the growth of non-hospital-based health facilities.

Accurate national employment data on health care employees by occupation are not available. Annual employment estimates are made by the National Center for Health Statistics, U.S. Department of Health, Education and Welfare, but there are doubts as to their accuracy. For example, an examination of Table 4 indicates that the estimated number of radiologic technicians has remained constant at 100,000 over the five-year period from 1968 through 1973. It is highly unlikely that the number employed in this occupation actually remained constant. Although the estimates of the National Center for Health Statistics may be the best figures available, they are often furnished by a self-serving group, such as the professional organization representing the employees of that occupation.

As indicated above, the hundreds of allied health occupations range in skill and training requirements from the college graduate down to those who, without a high school diploma, can be trained on the job within a few weeks to perform the functions of an occupation. There is no general agreement in the industry on the specific education and training requirements of each of the numerous occupations. For that matter, there are often significant differences in hiring-in practices for the same occupation within a limited geographic area. It is not uncommon for a hospital to require a high school education for a nurse's aide position, if it is possible to hire persons with that qualification, while another hospital in the same area does not. And if serious difficulties in hiring arise, the hospitals may consider lowering the educational requirement. There have been no studies to determine what the realistic education and training requirements are for all the health occupations.

Table 4 shows twenty allied health occupations that may be considered as potentially entry-level fields. We note that many hospitals may not agree completely with this selection. However, in our research over the past ten years with a large cross section of hospitals

Table 4. Estimated Employment in Selected Health Occupations
That Are Potentially Entry-Level

Occupation	1968		1971		1973	
	Number	Percent Distribution	Number	Percent Distribution	Number	Percent Distribution
Clinical laboratory technician and assistant	61,000	1.6	67,000	1.5	67,000	1.5
Dental assistant	95,000	2.6	114,000	2.5	116,000	2.6
Dental laboratory technician	27,000	0.7	31,150	0.7	32,000	0.7
Dietetic technician	6,000	0.2	7,000	0.2	23,000	0.5
Medical library clerk	6,000	0.2	4,100	0.1	4,100	0.1
Record technician	26,000	0.7	43,000	1.0	45,000	1.0
Nurse's aide	786,000	21.2	875,000	19.4	910,000	20.5
Home health aide	14,000	0.4	25,000	0.6	28,000	0.6
Occupational therapy aide	5,500	0.1	6,500	0.1	6,500	0.1
Optometric assistant	n.a.	–	5,000	0.1	5,000	0.1
Optometric technician	n.a.		1,000	0.02	1,000	0.02
Physical therapy assistant	8,000	0.2	9,000	0.2	8,100	0.2
Radiologic technician	100,000	2.7	100,000	2.2	100,000	2.2
Respiratory therapist	8,000	0.2	12,000	0.3	12,000	0.3
Health office services	275,000	7.4	300,000	6.7	300,000	6.7
Social work aide	1,500	0.04	4,300	0.1	4,300	0.1
Ambulance attendant[a]	n.a.	–	5,600	0.1	207,000	4.6
Animal technician	n.a.	–	n.a.	–	5,000	0.1
Electrocardiograph technician	7,000	0.2	9,500	0.2	9,500	0.2
Electroencephalograph technician	3,000	0.1	3,500	0.1	4,000	0.1
Total employees in selected occupations	1,429,000	38.5	1,622,650	36.1	1,887,500	42.2
Total active health employees	3,706,350	100.0	4,502,250	100.0	4,448,250	100.0

Source: National Center for Health Statistics, *Health Resources Statistics 1974; 1972-73; and 1969* (Rockville, Md.: U.S. Department of Health, Education and Welfare, Health Resources Administration, Public Health Service).

n.a. – not available.

[a]The figure in the 1971 column represents hospital employees in 1969. The 1973 figure covers all ambulance attendants, whether or not employed in hospitals.

and other health facilities, we have seen these occupations filled by persons with a minimum of education and very little on-the-job training; and there was no question about the level of their performance on the job. In general, it is our assumption that if it can be done in some hospitals, it probably can be done in many others.

Total employment in the health industry rose from 3.7 million in 1968 to 4.4 million in 1973, for an increase over the five-year period of 20 percent. As seen in Table 4, over the same five-year period the number of employees in entry-level occupations rose from 1.4 million to 1.9 million, an increase of about 25 percent; and employees in these occupations represented about 42 percent of the total health industry employment. If one excludes the figures for ambulance attendant because of the significant change in usage, the rise in employment in these entry-level occupations was 18 percent. Of this selected group of occupations, several experienced substantially large absolute and percentage increases: medical record technicians, laboratory technicians, dietetic technicians, nurse's aides, home health aides, social work aides, and respiratory therapists (inhalation therapists).

Institutions that employ allied health manpower can be divided into three principal categories: hospitals, ambulatory facilities, and nursing and rest homes. The changing nature of the kinds of health industry employers in a large sample of institutional health providers in Boston and Cambridge can be seen in Table 5. The health facilities represented in this table number over 200. In percentage terms these calculations for 1973 include 100 percent of all forty-four hospitals, 90 percent of all 121 nursing and rest homes, and 78 percent of all ninety-six ambulatory facilities.

During the five-year period 1968-1973 the number of health workers employed in hospitals of the sample area of Boston and Cambridge increased by 25.3 percent, while maintaining approximately 80 percent of total health facilities' employment. Nursing and rest homes over the same period showed a slight decrease of 1.7 percent in the number of health personnel employed. Employment in these facilities in 1973 represented only 12.1 percent of total health employment in the area. Ambulatory facilities showed the greatest percentage increase in employment, amounting to 98.3 percent from

1968 through 1973. Total health manpower employment during the 1968-1973 period for all health facilities in the sample area increased by 24.8 percent.

Comparable national estimates of health manpower employment by hospitals, ambulatory facilities, and nursing and rest homes are not available. However, some indication of the changing nature of the industry, and therefore of health manpower employment, can be seen from the indices of utilization of health facilities (see Table 6). Over the five-year period 1968-1973 the average length of stay in hospitals declined by 7.1 percent for the United States and by 2.6 percent for the Boston-Cambridge area. During the same period the hospital occupancy rate declined modestly for the United States and for the Boston-Cambridge area, for changes of −1.9 and −2.2 percent respectively. The most significant change occurred in the number of outpatient visits. Between 1968 and 1973 total outpatient visits in United States nonfederal hospitals increased by 56.0 percent. For the Boston-Cambridge area the comparable rise was only 31.4 percent. This is the area of health care that has shown the greatest growth and that has the greatest potential for long-run expansion.

During the last decade the United States has experienced a marked increase in the demand for health care. Although the public's demand for and utilization of physicians has certainly not decreased, there has been a very strong upward movement in the utilization of hospital ambulatory facilities for the delivery of primary health care, principally in the form of outpatient visits. The relatively recent shift in the geographic distribution of primary-care physicians, especially their movement away from low-income areas of large urban centers, has virtually forced residents of these areas to turn to ambulatory facilities − principally the outpatient departments of municipal hospitals − for their primary health care needs. Medicare and Medicaid have also been important contributing factors in this shift in the utilization of health care resources.

Recent national data on nursing home and rest home facilities are not available, but estimates for the period 1963 to 1971 indicate that such facilities increased rapidly. The number of these facilities is said to have risen by 32 percent, the number of the beds in the facilities by 111 percent. In general, occupancy rates of nursing and rest

Table 5. Employment in Health Facilities in Boston-Cambridge and Distribution of Employees by Type of Employer, 1968, 1971, and 1973.

| Type of Employer | 1968 | | 1971 | | 1973 | | Percent Change | | |
	Number of Employees	Percentage [a]	Number of Employees	Percentage [a]	Number of Employees	Percentage [a]	1968-1971	1971-1973	1968-1973
Hospitals	15,760	79.8	18,633	79.4	19,759	80.2	18.2	6.0	25.3
Nursing and rest homes	3,027	15.3	3,245	13.8	2,976	12.1	7.2	-8.3	-1.7
Ambulatory facilities	954	4.8	1,596	6.8	1,892	7.7	67.3	18.5	98.3
TOTAL	19,741	99.9	23,474	100.0	24,627	100.0	18.9	4.9	24.8

Source: Preliminary data, Center for Medical Manpower Studies (Boston: Northeastern University), June 1976.

[a] Percentages may not add to 100 because of rounding.

Table 6. Utilization of Short-term Nonfederal Hospitals in United States and in Boston-Cambridge, 1968, 1971, and 1973

	Percent Change, 1968-1971		Percent Change, 1971-1973		Percent Change, 1968-1973	
	United States	Boston-Cambridge	United States	Boston-Cambridge	United States	Boston-Cambridge
Number of hospitals	0.4	a	0.9	a	1.2	a
Average Length of stay	-4.8	-6.9	-2.5	4.6	-7.1	-2.6
Outpatient visits	30.0	19.0	20.6	10.4	56.0	31.4
Occupancy rate	-3.6	—	-1.7	-2.2	-1.9	-2.2

Source: Preliminary data, Center for Medical Manpower Studies.

[a] Boston-Cambridge had 29 short-term nonfederal hospitals in 1968 and 1971; in 1973 there were 30 such hospitals.

homes tend to be fairly high, and estimates place the rates in the vicinity of 95 percent.[2]

The substantial growth in nursing home and rest home facilities, plus the significant increase in the utilization of ambulatory facilities, suggests some basic changes in the requirements of allied health manpower. Significantly larger numbers of allied health manpower are being employed by new kinds of health providers. In many instances the roles of health manpower employed by these new institutions vary considerably from the past. Hiring-in requirements, job descriptions, and licensing and certification requirements are not yet set in concrete. Opportunities do exist for a variety of innovations that would allow entry-level health personnel to fill meaningful jobs while fulfilling the specific needs of the consuming public.

Current Pattern of Utilization

There are a number of important factors that affect the utilization of health care employees by hospitals, the major employers of the industry. One is the hiring-in standards for entry-level positions. As is relatively common in many industries, hospitals generally set a high school diploma as a minimum requirement for even the least skilled job in the health care structure of positions. This is not a uniform practice, but most hospitals use such a standard even where it is not clearly job-related, and the result is to exclude large numbers of the disadvantaged from the industry.

A second factor affecting the utilization of health care employees is the failure of the industry to utilize occupations in accordance with the education, training, and skills required of persons in those occupations. There is a substantial overlapping of functions among various occupations, from entry-level to highly skilled, with little if any effort to rationalize the occupational structure.

A third factor is the rigid qualifying requirements established by a growing number of occupations, under the guise of professionalism, through such means as licensing and certification. Such qualifying requirements have made both vertical and lateral mobility exceedingly difficult. In many instances the training and experience gained in one occupation are not counted toward the requirements of another related occupation.

The general result of these factors is that disadvantaged persons and members of ethnic minorities who have little education find it difficult to break into the industry; and when they do it is almost always at entry-level positions that turn out to be low-paying, dead-end jobs. And because of the practice of permitting or fostering the overlap of functions among occupations, persons in entry-level positions often find themselves performing relatively high-level functions without the higher pay or the higher job classification title. After years of experience on the job, the only way of getting a promotion is to leave the job and enter an institutional training program. In all these ways, the cards are stacked against the disadvantaged and minority-group members who have little education.

Hiring-in Standards

Not only are there no uniform nationwide hiring-in standards for entry-level positions in the health care industry, but there also is little information as to what the various standards are. In 1967 and 1968 a study was conducted in the Boston area[3] with the objective of assessing the hiring standards of selected health care occupations — as measured by a comparison of the required education, training, and work experience — with the actual duties and functions performed on the job by persons in those occupations. The basic information was obtained through structured questionnaires and interviews with administrators, personnel directors, and employees in twenty hospitals stratified by size and type. The sample of employees covered 524 workers in twenty-two allied health occupations. Detailed information was gathered on hiring requirements for each of the twenty-two occupations and on the actual job performance of the 524 employees, as well as on their professional and educational background. Information was also collected on some general characteristics of the occupations, such as promotional possibilities, on-the-job training, and the importance of professional certification.

The findings in this study confirmed the hypothesis that hiring-in standards established by hospitals were higher than needed for the duties performed, and that this fact resulted in serious difficulties to fill many allied health positions. The hiring-in standards for most occupations were generally established internally by the hospitals, either on a department or a general administrative basis. For the entry-level and middle-level occupations there was less uniformity among the hospitals than at the higher occupations, although the high school diploma was required by almost all hospitals even for the entry-level jobs. Not only did the hiring standards vary among the hospitals, but in some cases there were variations between departments in the same hospital as well.

At the middle-level and higher occupations one is more likely to find the employees organized into professional societies, which often are affiliated with a state or national organization. Many of these professional societies, as well as accrediting agencies, have some influence over entrance requirements for their respective organizations, and they continue to press for additional professional and educational preparation. In response to this pressure colleges, universities, and other educational institutions offer a variety of allied health training programs, but the costs and the entrance requirements are often too high to permit matriculation by the poor and the educationally deprived.

The 1967-1968 research indicated that few hospitals in the Boston area were prepared to admit that the hiring standards recommended by professional societies and accrediting agencies and adopted by the hospitals were too high. Most hospitals indicated that the basic factors and levels of their hiring standards were in effect for many years, sometimes over ten years. Most hospitals considered their hiring standards to be just right, even though the job content and duties of a number of occupations had changed substantially over time and there was a labor shortage in many occupations.

Despite the specific standards set by the Boston area hospitals, many employees who had been hired without meeting the educational requirements were performing satisfactorily on the job. The information from that research report indicates that a number of employees in specific entry-level occupations had completed less than four years of high school (see Table 7). Thirty percent of the

Table 7. Percentage of Persons in Sampled Occupations Having
Completed Specified Years of School

| | Years of School Completed | |
| | Eight Years or Less | One to Three Years |
Occupation	of Elementary School	of High School
Licensed practical nurse	2.0	4.0
(N = 54)		
Nurse's aide	2.0	30.0
(N = 51)		
EKG technician	–	–
(N = 31)		
EEG technician	–	10.0
(N = 11)		
Inhalation therapist	–	17.6
(N = 17)		
X-ray developing machine		
operator	11.1	22.2
(N = 9)		
Physical therapist aide	20.0	20.0
(N = 5)		
Occupational and manual		
therapist	–	7.1
(N = 14)		
Dietary aide	19.0	33.0
(N = 21)		
Psychiatric aide	7.6	15.4
(N = 26)		

Source: Morris A. Horowitz and Harold M. Goldstein, *Hiring Standards for
Paramedical Manpower* (Boston: Northeastern University, 1968).

sampled nurse's aides and thirty-three percent of the dietary aides
had completed no more than one to three years of high school, and
in a number of other entry-level occupations there were employees
who had no more than eight years of elementary school education.
A good deal of similarity was found in the educational background
of the X-ray technician, EKG, EEG, and inhalation therapy employees. Although occupational training for these classifications varies
from several months to twenty-four months, their formal education
followed a similar pattern: few have any college education, and a
number have less than four years of high school education. These are
rapidly growing health care occupations, and the opportunities for
persons with no training appear to be good.

The 1968 study of hiring standards of hospitals in the Boston area provides information on hiring and training practices of the U.S. Navy Hospital (Chelsea), which appears to be considerably more efficient than other hospitals. The Navy was very successful in training medical corpsmen in a shorter period than the civilian training and education institutions, while the education requirements were less restrictive. The Navy, for example, trained X-ray technicians in twelve months, while the other hospitals in the Boston area required twenty-four months of training. The Navy trained EEG and EKG technicians in four months, whereas the civilian hospitals required anywhere from seven to twelve months of training. The Navy trained all of its corpsmen in a sixteen-week basic course and then required the laboratory assistants to take twelve additional weeks of training (a total of less than seven months). All of the civilian hospitals included in the research project required between twelve and sixteen months of training for the laboratory assistants. A high school diploma was not required by the Navy, but it was a requirement in all the other hospitals included in the survey.

The findings seem to confirm that Navy-trained technicians were highly qualified and readily employed by the civilian hospitals. Approximately 85 percent of the Navy-trained laboratory personnel of the U.S. Navy Hospital were moonlighting in civilian hospitals.

The Problems of Overlapping Functions

The 1968 research on hiring standards in Boston area hospitals[4] analyzed twenty-two health occupations and found considerable similarities between various pairs of occupations in the functions performed. In some cases the differences in functions were slight, although the hiring-in standards differed significantly. Some hospitals used a single generic job title and designated specific job duties, while other hospitals used two distinct titles to cover similar duties. Frequently, broad differences in hiring standards could not be justified by the minor differences in the functions performed.

There is considerable overlap in the functions performed by licensed practical nurses (LPNs) and nurse's aides (NAs). There are eight functions on which NAs spend an average of 80 percent of their time; LPNs spend an average of 63.5 percent of their time on the same functions. The LPN is typically exposed to fifteen months or more of formal professional training after high school, whereas the aide receives only a few weeks of informal on-the-job training and in many cases has not finished high school.

The findings showed only a slight difference, if any, between the laboratory technologist and the laboratory technician; in general the distribution of their work-time among the different functions was about the same. However, the technologist is required to have considerably more education and training than the technician who is performing adequately at the same or similar tasks.

It would be of interest to compare in detail LPNs with NAs and hematology technologists with hematology technicians. The LPNs hold a high school diploma and are usually exposed to fifteen months of formal professional schooling; the NAs range from high school graduate to considerably less. The technologist has a bachelor of science or arts degree, while the technician may have an associate of arts degree, a high school diploma, or even less.

Licensed Practical Nurses and Nurse's Aides. The list of functions on Table 8 is a complete account of the tasks performed by LPNs and NAs, and all persons interviewed in these two occupations acknowledged that these functions occupied more than 95 percent of their work week. The functions were ranked in order of difficulty in accordance with the ratings by the consulting LPNs and NAs and are listed from the most simple function to the most complex. Several of the functions toward the bottom of the list (supposedly more difficult and requiring more experience and training) were performed by most LPNs and by a smaller, though significant, percentage of the nurse's aides. However, these functions occupied a relatively small percentage of LPN and NA time. A much greater percentage of LPN time is spent performing the easier tasks than is spent on the more difficult tasks.

Table 8. Percent of Total Working Time Spent on Various Functions
by LPNs and NAs, and Percentage Performing Each Function

Functions (ranked from easiest to most difficult)	LPN		NA	
	Percent of Total Working Time[a]	Percent Performing Function	Percent of Total Working Time[a]	Percent Performing Function
1. Cleaning rooms, beds; answering patients' calls	13.7	98.0	18.4	96.0
2. Washing and dressing body of deceased person	2.1	78.0	1.2	69.0
3. Recording food and fluid intake and output	5.1	93.0	6.7	100.0
4. Feeding patients	7.7	87.0	11.9	90.0
5. Performing routine lab work, such as urinalysis	1.4	46.0	1.8	55.0
6. Bathing, dressing patients; assisting patients in walking and turning	17.5	91.0	20.4	96.0
7. Tube feeding	2.2	78.0	0.7	29.0
8. Ordering drugs for patients	2.4	61.0	0.4	8.0
9. Taking and recording temperature, pulse, respiration rate	5.0	98.0	8.0	90.0
10. Taking and recording blood pressure	2.5	100.0	0.8	29.0
11. Applying compress, ice bag, hot water bottle	3.3	98.0	2.8	88.0
12. Giving enemas, douches, alcohol rubs, massages	5.4	94.0	5.8	84.0
13. Dressing wounds	2.6	96.0	0.7	25.0
14. Assembling and using such equipment as catheters, tracheotomy tubes, and oxygen suppliers	3.9	94.0	1.0	35.0
15. Observing patients and reporting adverse reactions to physicians or nurses	5.8	100.0	4.9	86.0
16. Administering specified medication and noting time and amount on patients' charts	10.0	87.0	0.5	12.0
17. Sterilizing equipment and supplies using germicides, sterilizer, or autoclave	1.5	46.0	5.4	65.0

Table 8 (cont).

18.Setting up IV equipment, discontinuing IV service	2.4	83.0	0.9	37.0
19.Setting up and using BIRD respirator	2.3	56.0	0.4	24.0
20.Research	0.1	4.0	–	–
21.Teaching	0.7	17.0	0.4	8.0
22.Supervisory work	1.1	17.0	2.8	8.0
23.Desk work	1.2	9.0	1.2	20.0
24.Intensive care unit	0.6	6.0	–	–

Source: Horowitz and Goldstein, *Hiring Standards for Paramedical Manpower.*

a May not add to 100 percent because of rounding.

As one would expect, the NAs spend considerable time on the simple or easy functions. Analysis of the first six "easy" functions (1 through 6) on Table 8 indicates that 84.3 percent of the NAs perform these functions, which take an average of 60.4 percent of their time. However, the LPNs also spend a significant amount of time on these functions; 82.2 percent of the LPNs perform these functions, and they spend an average of 47.5 percent of their time on them.

Analysis of the six "more difficult" functions (14 through 19) indicates that 77.7 percent of the LPNs perform these functions, and they spend an average of 25.9 percent of their time on them. In comparison, 43.2 percent of the NAs also perform these duties, spending an average of 13.1 percent of their time. Of the nurse's aides performing these functions, 33 percent had not completed high school, and none had received any prolonged on-the-job or professional training. The average NA in the sample had worked at the occupation for 6.6 years. This amount of on-the-job experience apparently gave the average NA sufficient capability to perform a large proportion of tasks also performed by the LPN.

The significant differences between the LPNs with their higher level of training, and NAs seem to rest on the following functions: tube feeding (7), ordering drugs for patients (8), taking and recording blood pressure (10), dressing wounds (13), assembling and using such equipment as catheters, tracheotomy tubes, and oxygen supplies (14), setting up and using BIRD respirators (19) and the most important and significant item, administering specific medications and noting the time and amount on the patients' charts (16). The majority of the LPNs perform all the above functions, whereas the majority of NAs do not. Despite this fact, the LPNs spend only 15.9 percent of their time on these seven functions, and the NAs spend 4.5 percent.

The LPNs spent well over 60 percent of their time on routine tasks that can be learned easily and quickly. Since the LPNs averaged about fifteen months of formal professional training beyond high school and since there appears to be a shortage in this occupation, the expenditure of time by the LPN on simple functions seems difficult to justify. The NA, with far less formal schooling and considerably less formal professional training, appears to be quite adequate in performing these less-skilled, though necessary, simple patient-care duties. In several of the twenty hospitals included in the study, the NAs performed all the functions of the LPN, despite the differences in professional and educational background.

Laboratory Personnel. For each of the six technologist occupations in the group of laboratory personnel, there was a counterpart technician in the same field, and both were asked the same questions regarding job functions. In only one of the six comparisons made (cytotechnologists and cytotechnicians) were substantial differences found in the time-function analysis. In the remaining five comparisons made, only minor differences were found in the distribution of work time over a given set of functions. For example, in comparing hematology technologists and technicians, analysis of the first six easy functions (1 through 6) indicates that 97 percent of the technologists spend 60 percent of their time on these functions, whereas 87 percent of the technicians spend an average of 67 percent of their time performing these functions (see Table 9). A review of six more difficult functions (7 through 12) indicates that 54 percent of the technologists spend an average of 22.4 percent of their time on these functions and that 35 percent of the technicians spend an average of 17.4 percent of their time on them. In most of the other compari-

Table 9. Percentage of Total Working Time Spent on Various Functions by Hematology Technologists and Technicians, and Percentage Performing Each Function

Functions (ranked from easiest to most difficult)	Technologist		Technician	
	Percentage of Total Working Time[a]	Percentage Performing Function	Percentage of Total Working Time[a]	Percentage Performing Function
1. Drawing capillary and venous bloods	8.9	100.0	8.0	91.3
2. Staining blood smears	5.7	100.0	6.5	91.3
3. Collecting blood specimens for laboratory	5.0	90.0	5.5	86.9
4. Performing routine tests – Hct, Hgb, WBC, etc.	19.9	100.0	28.4	100.0
5. Performing routine tests				
a. Bleeding time	3.1	90.0	2.1	69.6
b. Clotting time	2.8	90.0	2.9	69.6
c. Prothrombin time	3.4	90.0	3.2	56.5
6. Reading differentials	11.2	100.0	10.6	86.9
7. Performing RBC test	3.9	90.0	4.6	82.6
8. Performing petic counts	6.0	100.0	5.1	91.3
9. Performing advanced coagulation tests				
a. Serial Thrombin tests	1.6	40.0	0.7	34.8
b. Partial thromboplastin time	2.4	70.0	1.1	30.4
c. Euglobulin	0.7	20.0	0.3	13.0
d. Factor V-VIII-X assays	0.7	30.0	0.3	8.7
10. Reading Lupus Erythematosus slides	3.1	70.0	0.6	56.5
11. Staining and reading:				
a. Peroxidase stain	1.1	40.0	0.5	8.7
b. Alkaline phosphatase stain	1.1	40.0	0.7	17.4
12. Reading bone marrow slides	1.8	40.0	0.5	8.7
13. Research	0.1	10.0	2.0	17.4
14. Teaching	6.8	70.0	2.7	39.1
15. Supervisory work	2.2	30.0	1.1	30.4
16. Other	8.0	80.0	9.6	60.9

Source: Horowitz and Goldstein, "Employment and Utilization of Allied Medical Manpower in Hospitals," summary of *Hiring Standards for Paramedical Manpower* (Boston: Northeastern University, September 1968.)

[a] May not add to 100 percent because of rounding.

sons made the percentage of technologists and technicians performing the same functions was even closer.

The vast majority of technicians seem to perform the same tasks
as the technologists in their field, but far more time and effort is devoted to the education and professional training of the technologists.
The technician, with a good deal less education and professional
training, is performing satisfactorily on the job.

Of the forty-eight technologists included in the 1968 study of
hiring standards in the Boston area, 77.2 percent had a bachelor's degree, 5.5 percent a master's degree, and 3.9 percent an associate of
arts degree; over 86 percent of the technologists had at least one of
these degrees. Of the ninety-eight technicians, only 2.0 percent had a
bachelor's degree, none a master's degree, and 5.2 percent an associate of arts degree. Thus, only 7.2 percent of the technicians had a
bachelor's or associate of arts degree; a majority had no more than a
high school education.

4

The Implications of Licensing and Certification

There is no question but that the physician is the head of the medical care team, and many groups in the health care industry try to emulate the effectiveness of the organization of the physician. Over the past several years numerous professional societies have been founded to represent specific occupations or occupational groups of allied health manpower. The avowed goals of these organizations are to improve the quality of personnel in a specific field and to raise the standards of the profession. One of the common means of attaining these goals is by having the government license the occupation or certify the employee.

The general purpose of a licensed occupation or profession was to protect the consumer from fraud and from incompetent personnel and to provide the general public with a degree of security that a licensed practitioner possessed some acceptable level of knowledge in the field. The process provided the licensee with a government certification to the public at large that he met certain standards, and this in turn gave a greater degree of geographic mobility. From the point of view of the labor market, licensing had the direct effect of limiting entrance to the profession, and it indirectly affected the earning capacity of members of the profession.

Licensing in the Health Industry

In the health care field licensing has generally been imposed by individual occupational and professional groups, rather than by consumer groups or agencies of government. It would be naive to believe that health care groups pressuring for licensing of their occupation or profession are unaware of or unconcerned with the implications of their activities on the supply of manpower for their profession. Licensed professions are given some protection from competition by outsiders.

According to one student of this phenomenon,[1] licensing laws have the following effects: they increase the cost of entry to the occupation; they generally produce favorable income effects for the licensees; they usually result in higher age of entry into the trade; and they usually require longer periods of schooling than are strictly necessary for acquiring the skills and knowledge relevant to the practice of the craft.

An alternative to licensure is certification. Health performers who meet certain set standards can be certified. Performers who do not meet the standard are not certified, although they can and do perform the same health service. Because the certification process is less restrictive, it is referred to as "permissive licensing."

Although there has been a marked increase in licensing among the allied health professions, the nature of the industry and of employment in the industry has limited the impact of licensing upon the labor market. The principal problem is that enforcement of licensing and certification requirements in a hospital setting is very difficult. When a medical service in a hospital has to be performed, someone — presumably qualified, regardless of credentials or occupation — is assigned to perform the service. Numerous categories of allied health personnel overlap in the performance of medical tasks, and the decisions of physicians and supervisors as to who is to perform what function are often sheer chance. As indicated above, various nursing functions are performed by entry-level nurse's aides as well as by licensed practical nurses and registered nurses. Such a practice makes it almost impossible for a licensed profession to carve out a set of functions for itself and to exclude all others from performing these functions. And often it is not possible to determine which of the following occupational classifications performs in the most acceptable fashion: the certified personnel, the licensed personnel, or the entry-level personnel who have had on-the-job experience.

Ballenger and Estes outline the disadvantages of the licensure process:

First of all, it provides no real guarantee of the quality of professional acceptance of the group licensed. Regarding the individual licensees, it is questionable whether substantial quality control can be exerted by an administrative board having at best only intermittent contacts with the practitioners whom it licenses.

Secondly, licensure requires a description of the activities and functions of the designated professions. If these are precisely delineated, new tasks or responsibilities cannot be assumed without a change in the law, which may entail prolonged and costly delays. If they are loosely or vaguely defined, non-uniform interpretation of the boards of the professions, with consequent legal uncertainties, is the result.

Thirdly, licensure can become a weapon with which a given profession, jealously guarding its boundaries against encroachment, can frustrate reasonable accretion of its pre-empted duties by other groups over time. In addition, as new functions emerge through technologic and organizational changes, these may overlap jurisdictions and become a matter of legal dispute. Characteristics such as these have the effect of inhibiting innovation at a time when it is sorely needed and have led to suggestions not only that licensure should not be pursued for new health professions but also that the existing licensure structure should be abolished.[2]

Ballenger, a lawyer, and Estes, a physician, are addressing themselves here to the licensure of allied health manpower, when in fact their comments, which cannot be strongly refuted, can be applied to their own professions. In particular, the licensure laws governing physicians are obviously the model at which all other allied health groups look with envy. Once a physician is given a license to practice medicine, it is for life, since the instances of this license being revoked for justifiable reasons are extremely rare. And for a person to practice medicine without a license is a serious offense.

Table 10. Percent of Certified Employees in Selected Health Care
Occupations

Occupation	Percent Certified
Occupational therapist	86.0
Physical therapist	67.0
Orthotics and prosthetics worker	33.0
X-ray technician	40.0
Medical social worker	50.0
Psychiatric social worker	75.0
Medical librarian	9.0
Medical records librarian	12.0
Dental hygienist	100.0
Dental assistant	4.0
Dental technician	24.0
Clinical laboratory technician	43.0
Dietician	40.0
Inhalation therapist	5.0
Electroencephalograph technician	1.0

Source: Harry I. Greenfield (with the assistance of Carol A. Brown), *Allied
Health Manpower: Trends and Prospects* (New York: Columbia
University Press, 1969).

The comments of Forgotson and Roemer can be applied equally
to all professions, but especially to physicians and allied health personnel:

Current professional licensure laws do not generally recognize that
development of new information renders a person's initial qualifications obsolete unless they are upgraded periodically by continuing
education . . . . The licensure process makes no provision to guard
against educational obsolescence.[3]

New techniques, new technologies, and scientific discoveries in the
health industry make medical knowledge obsolete at a very rapid
rate.

The licensing policy for the hundreds of allied health occupations
varies from state to state. The problem of defining trends in the certification or licensure of the various allied health occupations is further complicated by the paucity of national data. Gathering such
data has been the responsibility of the National Center for Health

Table 11.   Health Personnel Required to be Licensed in All States
and the District of Columbia, 1973

Dental hygienists	Physicians (M.D.)
Dentists	Physicians (D.O.)
Embalmers	Podiatrists
Environmental health engineers	Practical nurses
Optometrists	Registered nurses
Pharmacists	Veterinarians
Physical therapists	

Source: National Center for Health Statistics, *Health Resource Statistics
1974*, p. 537.

Statistics of the U.S. Department of Health, Education and Welfare.
However, as noted by many, including the American Public Health
Association, this task has hardly been fulfilled adequately. Data
from *Health Resources Statistics 1965* indicate the approximate levels of certification in those allied health occupations for which information was available.

As noted by Greenfield and Brown, these estimates can be very
misleading. For example, 35 percent of the medical librarians have
professional library training, yet only 9 percent have been certified
(see Table 10). Among clinical laboratory technicians, 43 percent
are certified; an additional 5 percent, however, have higher educational qualifications than are required for certification.

According to the National Center for Health Statistics there are
thirty-five health occupations that are licensed, but only thirteen are
licensed in all states and the District of Columbia[4] (see Table 11).
Of the remaining health occupations that are licensed, there are eight
that can be considered as potentially entry-level positions (see Table
12). By entry-level positions, the authors mean those classifications
in which persons with no specialized training are hired and then are
trained on the job in a short time to perform the work of that position satisfactorily.

Since 1966 there has been a proliferation of licensed and certified
health groups that in some ways created an administrative nightmare
for hospital administrators, chiefs of services, and directors of hospital services. Flexible personnel policies are needed in hospitals to en-

Table 12. Entry-Level Health Personnel Licensure Status, 1973

Occupation	Number of States Requiring License
Dental laboratory technician	1
Occupational therapy assistant	1
Optholomic laboratory technician	2
Physical therapist assistant	15
Psychiatric aide	3
Radiologic technologist	4
Inhalation therapist	1
Sanitary technician	1

Source: National Center for Health Statistics, *Health Resource Statistics 1974*, pp. 537-540.

sure prompt and efficient services. Licensing and certification have, to some extent, limited upward mobility and made many entry-level positions dead-end jobs. These restrictions must be loosened if there is to be full utilization of competent entry-level personnel. The development and increased use of education equivalency and proficiency examinations could extend substantially the job opportunities for entry-level personnel without compromising the quality of health care available to the public.

Projects Aimed at Affecting the Problems of Licensing

Over the last decade there have been a number of research, development, and demonstration projects that have aimed at studying, alleviating, or eliminating this licensing and certification problem. Most of these projects have been funded by the federal government; some have been completely funded by hospitals.

Restructuring Paramedical Occupations

The demonstration project, entitled *Restructuring Paramedical Occupations* was funded by the Manpower Administration of the

U.S. Department of Labor and was completed in 1972.[5] This project was conducted at a municipal hospital in the Boston area over the three-year period from 1969 to 1972. Because the hospital was under the jurisdiction of the state civil service system and because the project was experimenting with categories of medical functions across occupational lines, the researchers asked for and received the cooperation of the Massachusetts Civil Service Commission. Through the cooperation of the hospital administration and the civil service commission, additional job classifications were established to avoid the barriers created by licensing and to permit upward job mobility.

Upgrading NAs to LPNs through a Work-Study Program

A report entitled "Upgrading Nurses Aides to LPNs through a Work-Study Program"[6] outlines a project funded by the Manpower Administration, U.S. Department of Labor and the U.S. Office of Education in the Department of Health, Education and Welfare. This project, sponsored by the AFL-CIO in New York City, demonstrated that many applicants who usually would not be accepted in LPN training programs can be successfully trained to function at the LPN level. Four hundred fifty entry-level aides were selected out of 2,800 applicants on the basis of attendance records, achievement test scores, and job evaluations. The aides selected were considered to be highly motivated students. The hypothesis tested was whether these highly motivated students, who had received low achievement scores, could be successful after being provided with remedial education.

The work-study program lasted fourteen months. Students worked twenty hours per week at their normal work assignments, for which they earned their regular rate of pay; they also spent twenty-five hours per week in LPN schooling, for which they earned a training stipend. Income from the stipend plus the twenty hours of regular work was equal to an aide's normal full-time income.

The traditional training program for LPNs was supplemented with material to compensate for the students' prolonged absence from traditional schooling, including a six-week remedial program in mathematics and reading, as well as counseling, individual tutoring, and intensive review sessions to prepare for the LPN licensing examination.

Of the 422 people who completed the program 385, including a substantial number of those designated as highly motivated, passed the state board examinations. Supervisors' evaluations of LPNs who completed the experimental program showed that by and large they were as good as or better than the LPNs who had completed the regular program. The project has since been expanded to determine whether similar procedures via the work-study route can be adapted to upgrade LPNs to RNs.[7]

The Eastern Maine Medical Center

As mentioned above, hospital administrators and chiefs of services have great capacity to find personnel to provide required medical functions in their own institutions, irrespective of externally imposed licensure requirements. Rural and sparsely populated areas of the nation have had difficulty in staffing their medical facilities, and rigid adherence to the requirements of the licensed and registered classifications could make it almost impossible to provide satisfactory service. A good example of just how medical providers accommodate their needs is illustrated by the entry-level programs established at the Eastern Maine Medical Center in Bangor, Maine.

The Eastern Maine Medical Center is a 360-bed short-term private nonprofit hospital located in a sparsely populated rural area. The hospital serves the medical needs of patients located from 100 miles south of Bangor to the Canadian border, 200 miles north. Since 1969 this hospital has conducted an in-service training program to provide upgrading opportunities for its allied health personnel. It currently has in-service training programs for (1) nursing assistants, (2) senior nursing assistants, (3) nursing technicians, (4) senior nursing technicians, and (5) LPNs by waiver. The entry-level position is the nursing assistant, and the other positions are used as steps in the promotion ladder. In addition, the nursing in-service education department is also involved in a "co-op" on-the-job training program for high school students.

The data in Table 13 indicate the impact of these in-service and on-the-job training programs for entry-level allied health occupations. Functions and tasks were placed in groups (1 through 5) and ranked in order of difficulty or complexity. Group 1 represents the easiest functions, whereas Group 3 represents the more sophisticated or complex medical functions. Groups 4 and 5 are administrative and pediatric functions that do not necessarily indicate degree of difficulty.

The movement from nursing assistant to senior nursing assistant to nursing technician to senior nursing technician makes a logical progression during in-service training. In general, a greater percentage of performers spends increasing amounts of time on the more sophisticated functions as they proceed through the levels of training and up the promotion ladder.

It should be noted that the Eastern Maine Medical Center proceeded with this continuing upgrading program for entry-level health occupations with its own funds. No local, state, or federal assistance was used; it apparently did not occur to Medical Center officials to seek outside funding. Further, the administrative personnel of the hospital assumed that their training and upgrading efforts were probably quite common among hospitals, which is certainly not the case. Relatively few hospitals in the United States are involved with this kind or any kind of in-service training and education for entry-level personnel.

The University of Chicago Hospitals and Clinics

The AFL-CIO project in New York City mentioned above was aiming to provide in-service education and training in order to bring entry-level personnel up to the level of LPN. A hospital that has succeeded in bringing its entry-level employees to the RN level deserves special mention. In 1971 the University of Chicago Hospitals and Clinics employed 2,300 persons, of whom approximately 10 percent were considered to be holding dead-end, low-paying jobs. Despite union representation for twenty-six years, these employees had a general feeling that they were being denied advancement. After a

Table 13. Percentage of Total Working Time Spent on Groups of Functions (1) and Average Percentage Performing Within Each Group of Functions (2) at the Eastern Maine Medical Center

Groups of functions (ranked from easiest to most difficult)	Registered Nurse (1)[a]	(2)	Senior Nursing Technician (1)[a]	(2)	Nursing Technician (1)[a]	(2)	Senior Nursing Assistant (1)[a]	(2)	Nursing Assistant (1)[a]	(2)
Group 1 (functions 1-18)	20.5	80.0	42.5	94.0	44.9	95.0	48.8	93.2	49.5	90.0
Group 2 (functions 19-30)	16.0	84.0	38.5	96.0	34.3	93.7	31.5	89.9	30.0	68.7
Group 3 (functions 31-47)	25.2	86.0	12.6	64.0	10.8	65.0	10.0	56.6	12.1	46.2
Group 4 (functions 48-63)	38.3	88.0	6.4	40.0	7.4	40.0	9.7	56.6	8.4	43.7
Group 5 (functions 64-69)	0.1	20.0	—	—	2.0	12.5	—	—	—	—
Number of personnel included in study sample	5		5		3		8		3	

Source: Preliminary data, Center for Medical Manpower Studies.

[a] May not add to 100 because of rounding.

wildcat strike in 1969, task force groups were formed in each of the three major departments of the hospital: nursing, dietary, and general services. As a result, by February 1971 basic remedial programs had been started along with career ladders for entry-level health personnel (see Figure 1).[8]

The four principles of this Career Mobility Program were:

1. Education must be tied directly and specifically to mobility.
2. Each program should start where the individual is in the career mobility sequence of the job progression.
3. Training at one level should contain core knowledge and skill development that is applicable to the next level.
4. There is a need to link together educational components of the system in order to utilize scarce teaching resources effectively.[9]

Institutional Licensing

Over the last decade a number of students of the health care licensing issue have begun to advocate the elimination of governmental and professional licensing for most categories of allied health personnel. Nathan Hershey, one such advocate, has suggested an expansion of the existing state and professional licensing programs for health providers (hospitals, extended care facilities, and ambulatory facilities) in order to have more direct controls over employed allied health manpower. He makes a reasonable distinction between health professionals who practice their trade in a rather independent fashion — such as physicians and dentists — and such health personnel as registered nurses, therapists, and health technologists and technicians, who almost always perform their services under the institutional umbrella of a health care provider. Hershey makes the cogent point that "when individuals seek services today at a health institution, with regard to nurses, physical therapists and other aides, they rely on the institution to determine the qualifications and capability of such personnel. They assume that the institution has evaluated the personnel it employs to act on its behalf."[10] Institutional licensure would allow health providers to establish medical functions and job descriptions with the approval of an appropriate state agency, so

Figure 1. Career Ladders, University of Chicago Hospitals and Clinics

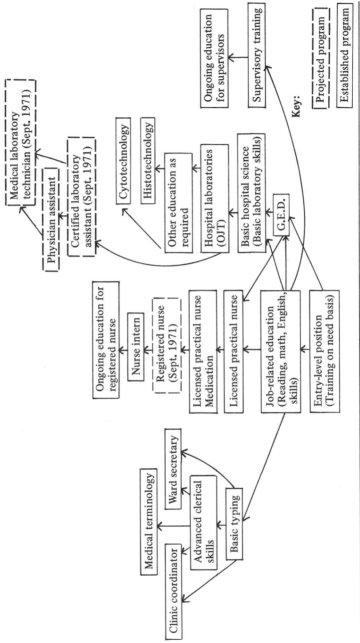

Source: Sally Holloway and Robert G. Holloway, "The Development of a Program of Career Mobility in Hospitals," Paper presented at the American Hospital Association convention (Chicago: AHA, August 1971), p. 25.

that there would be no need for individual licensure by professional groups or governmental agencies. Direct responsibility would be placed upon a provider of health care to allocate medical functions among its various categories of allied health manpower. Equal responsibility would be borne by state regulatory agencies to ensure that proper and qualified health manpower were being utilized by all health providers in an atmosphere that would provide the consumers with some assurance that they were being served by qualified personnel.

In order to clear up some of the misconceptions concerning institutional licensure, Nathan Hershey and Walter S. Wheeler, under the auspices of the California Hospital Association, published a very useful question-and-answer booklet entitled "Health Personnel Regulation in the Public Interest — QA on Institutional Licensure." This pamphlet clears up some erroneous notions concerning institutional licensure.[11]

Q. Would each health institution issue licenses to its employees?

A. No. Because only health institutions would be directly regulated by the government, licenses would be required only of the employing institutions, not of the individual health workers within the institutions.

Q. Would each health institution be required to have exactly the same job descriptions and qualifications?

A. No. Illustrative job descriptions established by the institutional licensing agency would be in the nature of guides, rather than mandated requirements. Actual job descriptions and related qualifications would be developed in line with the organizational need of the institution.

Q. Would more flexible job descriptions help in the distribution of health manpower?

A. Yes. Depending upon the availability of personnel within a locality, a health institution might revise job descriptions which are unrealistic in terms of the area's available health personnel, and through modifying its current plan for delivery of health service, better utilize the human resources in the local manpower pool.

Q. What would a health institution do if it found that there were insufficient personnel with certain qualifications available to perform necessary tasks and functions?

A. What health institutions frequently do now: establish an in-service training program or a program with a local educational institution, to develop new personnel with the skills in short supply. Alternatively, an institution could provide programs of continuing education to permit present health workers to acquire the necessary skills. This is precisely the process that led to the many new categories of health workers coming on the scene.

The four questions and answers noted above are only a sample of the issues noted in the brochure. Institutional licensure does seem to present a viable alternative to the present maze and inefficiencies of the federal, state, local, and professional licensure regulation.

In July 1972 a project was undertaken by W. Randolph Tucker and Burtchaell G. Wetterau at the Rush-Presbyterian-St. Luke's Medical Center in Chicago, to evaluate the feasibility and methodology of utilizing the in-house credentialing capability of hospitals as a supplement or alternative to existing means of credentialing allied health manpower. Only nonlicensed personnel functioning in dependent roles were included in this study.[12] The following thirteen functional areas were covered.

1. Biomedical engineering
2. Clinical laboratories
3. Dietetics and nutrition
4. Medical records
5. Occupational therapy
6. Physical therapy
7. Specialized rehabilitation therapy
8. Radiology and nuclear medicine
9. Respiratory therapy
10. Surgical services
11. Transfusion and IV therapy
12. Speech and hearing
13. Other

The study covered nineteen hospitals employing a total of 22,215 persons. In these hospitals 3,329 health performers were surveyed; of these, 2,366, or 71.1 percent, were employed in a classification for which a formal credentialing mechanism existed (see Table 14). Using these 2,366 as the universe the study found that almost 60 percent had formal credentials and 40 percent were employed in the same classifications without formal credentials.[13]

Some of the more significant findings of this study were –

1. The basic problems surrounding institutional licensure were technical, fiscal, political, and emotional.

2. There was a significant discrepancy among the hospitals' conceptions of titles, functions, tasks, and definitions of the numerous allied health roles.

3. Overlapping of functional and task performance among numerous levels of allied health manpower was rampant. A significant number of tasks were performed by numerous categories of allied health manpower with varying levels of education and experience.

In general the study concluded that –

1. The elements of institutional licensure would appear to be generally acceptable to a broad spectrum of hospital administration reprooontativoo.

2. Many institutions would have misgivings about various practical aspects of institutional licensure.

3. The political, technical, and emotional problems involved in implementing institutional licensure made it infeasible at that time.[14]

Although this study of the feasibility of promoting institutional licensure was considered by its authors something of a failure, one can look at a few other factors that are indicated in the study. The first is that 40 percent of those studied were performing (apparently successfully) without certification in categories for which a formal credentialing mechanism existed. This may mean that the credentialing process is not directly related to ability to perform on the job and is being used as a mechanism to limit the supply of persons in the classification. A second factor is that institutional licensure seemed infeasible because of the opposition of the credentialing organizations. A number of the personnel categories listed in Table 14 can be considered as entry-level positions. The credentialing mechanism can be a barrier to these entry-level jobs.

Table 14. Personnel in Categories for Which a Formal
Credentialing Mechanism Exists

Allied Health Personnel Survey
November 1972

Category	Total Number	Number with Formal Credentials	Number without Formal Credentials
Blood bank technologist	42	17	25
Cytotechnologist	33	28	5
Histologic technician	70	49	21
Laboratory assistant	110	21	89
Medical laboratory technician	301	44	257
Medical technologist	468	387	81
Biochemistry technologist	35	32	3
Microbiology technologist	14	13	1
Hematology technologist	32	31	1
Dietitian[a]	114	107	7
Medical records administrator	32	31	1
Medical records technician	39	22	17
Occupational therapist	45	44	1
Occupational therapy assistant	9	3	6
Physical therapist[b]	86	80	6
Nuclear medicine technician [c]	20	6	14
Nuclear medicine technologist	28	22	6
Radiation therapy technologist	28	21	7
Radiologic technologist	314	294	20
Respiratory therapist	80	46	34
Respiratory therapy technician	174	57	117
Pulmonary technologist	1	–	1
Audiologist	4	4	–
Speech pathologist[d]	21	16	5
Operating room technician	196	17	179
Clinical perfusionist	2	1	1
Music therapist	1	1	–
Recreation therapist	6	1	5
Cardio-respiratory technician	33	1	32
Electroencephalograph technician	27	6	21
Orthoptic technician	1	1	–
TOTAL	2,366	1,403(59.3%)	963(40.7%)

Source: W. Randolph Tucker and Burtchaell G. Wetterau, *Credentialing
Health Personnel by Licensed Hospitals: the Report of a Study of
Institutional Licensure* (Chicago: Rush-Presbyterian-St. Luke's
Medical Center, February 1975), I:19.

Table 14. Continued

a Included in this category are 19 dietitians, registered by the American Dietetics Association, who were classified as "nutritionists."

b The six physical therapists without formal credentials are awaiting the state of Illinois registration exam.

c Nuclear medicine technician is a locally designated term. In consideration of the credentialing mechanism, technicians have been listed separately from technologists.

d Included in this category is a speech pathologist certified by the American Speech and Hearing Association, who was classified as a "speech correction therapist."

5

Restructuring Allied Health Occupations

We have indicated some of the general problems affecting the utilization of allied health personnel. One study comments on this phenomenon as follows:

One of the most important barriers to optimum utilization of allied health personnel is the extreme specialization of workers and the overly rigid separation between types of workers. This is reinforced by professional organizations of each type of worker, by separate training facilities, and by outdated laws and anachronistic customs. Among the consequences of this malutilization are deadend occupations, high turnover rates, job dissatisfaction, and higher operating costs.[1]

These barriers to optimum utilization of personnel have been particularly burdensome to the disadvantaged and members of ethnic minorities. The ports of entry to the industry that are open to these persons are usually low-paying dead-end jobs, and opportunities for advancement are very limited because of the rigid institutional barriers that have been fostered by professional organizations and accepted by administrators of hospitals.

Is it possible to make substantial changes in the system so that more job and promotion opportunities are available to the disadvantaged and to others who may come into the industry at entry-level jobs? In June 1969 a research and demonstration project was undertaken at a single hospital to determine whether the system could be changed.[2] It was recognized that success or failure in one hospital did not guarantee similar results for the whole industry. However, an important aim of the project was to develop recommendations that would be applicable to and implemented by many hospitals across the nation. With that in mind every effort was made to select a hospital that was somewhat representative of many others in the United States and that was prepared to cooperate in the research and demonstration effort.

The principal objectives of this project were —

1. to study and analyze the hiring-in requirements and duties and functions of allied health personnel in a single hospital;

2. to recommend changes to restructure health occupations and to improve the utilization of health manpower in that hospital;

3. to evaluate the successes and failures involved in the implementation of the recommendations;

4. to measure changes in quantity and quality of medical services resulting from the implementation of the recommendations; and to relate changes in service to such factors as changes in hiring-in standards, job duties and functions, and job structure.

It may be noted that special emphasis was placed on the expansion of job opportunities in entry-level positions.

An additional objective of the project was to study and analyze the problems encountered when a hospital introduces basic changes in its occupational structure. Such an analysis could help determine whether obstacles to implementation are unique to a specific hospital or are basic to all hospitals and other health providers. After the recommendations were made, the project's main effort was to aid the hospitals in implementing the recommendations and in maintaining a detailed account of the ease and difficulties encountered in the efforts at implementation. Implementation by this hospital could have a demonstration effect for numerous other hospitals and health providers that have the same or similar problems with effective utilization of allied health manpower. Further, such findings could highlight the legal, institutional and other barriers that have impeded the recommended changes at this hospital and are likely to impede similar changes attempted by other health providers.

The hospital selected for the study was The Cambridge Hospital, a municipal hospital in the city of Cambridge, Massachusetts.[3] It appeared to be a fairly representative hospital, and the administrator, the professional organizations, and the unions offered their cooperation in the project. This cooperation in no way implied that all relationships in the hospital were harmonious. They were not. The Cambridge Hospital faced problems similar to those of most hospitals in the country, and as a municipal hospital many of its problems were compounded. However, it was felt that if significant changes in the utilization of manpower could be made in such an environment, they surely could be duplicated in other institutions.

The study in The Cambridge Hospital covered a wide range of health occupations, as shown in Table 15. The findings here more or less duplicated the findings of the earlier study, *Hiring Standards for Paramedical Personnel*, but much more detailed information became available. One of the key findings was that there was a substantial amount of overlapping of functions performed by registered nurses (RNs), licensed practical nurses (LPNs), nurse's aides (NAs), and orderlies, and a smaller amount of overlap between other health occupations. An examination of the information for the nursing occupations points up the problems of the inefficient utilization of allied health personnel.

Almost all persons in the four nursing occupations performed the easiest functions. For example, "straightening up and cleaning patients' immediate furniture" was performed by all of the LPNs and orderlies and by over 90 percent of the RNs and NAs. Despite the simplicity of this function, the RNs and LPNs spent a larger percentage of their time on it than did the NAs and orderlies. Among those who performed the function, the following average times were spent:

RNs, 7.5 percent;
LPNs, 9.2 percent;
NAs, 6.0 percent;
Orderlies, 4.9 percent.

Examination of a more difficult function, demanding more skill and training, "discontinuing IV service," shows that the distribution of work is not much different than for the very simple functions. This difficult function was performed by all LPNs, almost all the RNs, and slightly more than half the NAs and orderlies. Among those who performed this difficult function, the following average times were spent:

RNs, 5.1 percent;

LPNs, 5.1 percent;

NAs, 1.9 percent;

Orderlies, 2.7 percent.

Table 16 shows the distribution of functions among the four nursing occupations in the different nursing departments. The first category, general nursing, summarizes all the departments: one notes

Table 15. Personnel Interviewed at The Cambridge Hospital,
by Occupation

Occupation	Number Interviewed	Number Employed	Percentage Interviewed
Registered nurse	45	51	88.2
Licensed practical nurse	10	17	58.8
Nurse's aide	28	31	90.3
Orderly	8	8	100.0
Ward secretary	6	9	66.7
Surgical technician	7	8	87.5
Psychiatric attendant	7	7	100.0
X-ray technician	12	12	100.0
EKG technician	1	1	100.0
Inhalation therapy technician	4	4	100.0
Neighborhood health worker	1	1	100.0
Laboratory technician:			
Hematology technician	2	2	100.0
Blood bank technician	2	3	66.7
Bacteriology technician	2	2	100.0
Cytology technician	1	1	100.0
Histology technician	2	2	100.0
Urinanlysis and parasitology technician	1	1	100.0
Chemistry technician	2	2	100.0
Administrative and supervisory personnel	38	42	90.5
TOTAL	179	204	87.7

Source: Goldstein and Horowitz, *Restructuring Paramedical Occupations* (Boston: Northeastern University, 1972), I:19.

Table 16. Average Percentage of Time Spent on Three Groups of Functions[a]

	RN	LPN	NA	Orderly
I. *General Nursing* [b] (summary of Groups II-VII) Groups of Functions (ranked from easiest to most difficult)				
Group 1 (1-18)	24.7	31.5	40.8	40.8
Group 2 (19-30)	26.3	28.2	38.2	26.1
Group 3 (31-47)	20.3	22.5	6.4	15.6
Miscellaneous	28.5	17.7	14.5	17.1
II. *Surgical Unit* Groups of Functions (ranked from easiest to most difficult)				
Group 1 (1-18)	21.6	28.0	39.4	36.7
Group 2 (19-30)	31.3	33.7	41.9	29.1
Group 3 (31-47)	22.8	17.2	7.9	16.5
Miscellaneous	24.3	21.1	10.7	17.8
III. *Medical Unit* Groups of Functions (ranked from easiest to most difficult)				
Group 1 (1-18)	23.4	27.4	36.3	39.0
Group 2 (19-30)	27.4	28.9	47.2	27.7
Group 3 (31-47)	20.6	28.6	4.5	15.2
Miscellaneous	28.4	15.0	12.0	18.2
IV. *Pediatrics Unit* Groups of Functions (ranked from easiest to most difficult)				
Group 1 (1-18)	32.8	42.9	51.7	—[c]
Group 2 (19-30)	23.7	21.5	24.2	—
Group 3 (31-47)	17.6	12.7	7.4	—
Miscellaneous	26.3	22.8	16.7	—
V. *Labor and Delivery Unit* Groups of Functions (ranked from easiest to most difficult)				
Group 1 (1-18)	19.4	—	35.4	—
Group 2 (19-30)	15.4	—	25.9	—
Group 3 (31-47)	17.3	—	7.5	—
Miscellaneous	37.9	—	31.2	—

Table 16. Continued

VI. Emergency Unit
   Groups of Functions (ranked from
   easiest to most difficult)

Group 1 (1-18)	–	39.1	–	43.2
Group 2 (19-30)	–	23.6	–	21.4
Group 3 (31-47)	–	20.2	–	20.5
Miscellaneous	–	17.0	–	14.7

VII. Out-Patient Department
   Groups of Functions (ranked from
   easiest to most difficult)

Group 1 (1-18)	26.5	–	49.5	–
Group 2 (19-30)	24.3	–	30.5	–
Group 3 (31-47)	21.3	–	10.2	–
Miscellaneous	27.8	–	9.7	–

Source: Goldstein and Horowitz, *Restructuring Paramedical Occupations,*
    I:48-49.

[a] This table presents the average of all performers' time, whether they performed the function or not, and therefore figures should add up to approximately 100 percent. Figures were adjusted proportionately to add up to approximately 100 percent because there was no reason to believe that a disproportionate bias occurred in estimation of time for each group as a whole.

[b] This section is a summary of all specific units: Surgical, Medical, Pediatrics, Labor and Delivery, Emergency and Out-Patient Department. The RN column also includes intensive care unit, recovery room, and "floats."

[c] Dashes indicate that no individuals in the category were interviewed in that department.

that all four of the occupations perform both the easy and the difficult nursing functions.

From these statistical data the following conclusions were reached:

1. There was a great deal of overlap in the performance of various functions irrespective of the degree of difficulty and the education, formal or otherwise, of various categories of allied health personnel (RNs, LPNs, NAs, and orderlies) at The Cambridge Hospital.

2. Although the more difficult functions were performed more by personnel with higher levels of professional training and knowledge, the less-skilled allied health employees did perform these functions more than occasionally.

3. The more highly-skilled persons spent large blocks of their time on functions they and most other authorities considered to be well below their technical capabilities.

4. All four of these health occupations (RNs, LPNs, NAs, and orderlies) performed most of their high level functions during shifts other than the day shift. This was especially true of the LPNs, NAs, and orderlies. During the shift from 11:00 p.m. to 7:00 a.m., RNs, LPNs, NAs, and orderlies were called upon to perform functions that only physicians or RNs would normally perform during the day.

Supporting these findings are the conclusions of a progress report of the Social Development Corporation.

(a) With reference to these 51 items, at least one Registered Nurse, Licensed Practical Nurse, and Nurse Aide are performing identical tasks in 14 cases (27.4 percent).

(b) In 45 of 51 cases (88.2 percent) Registered Nurses and Licensed Practical Nurses are performing the identical tasks.

(c) In 18 of 51 cases (35.3 percent) Registered Nurses and the Nurse Aide are performing identical tasks.

(d) In 19 of 51 cases (37.2 percent) Licensed Practical Nurses and the Nurse Aide are performing identical tasks.[4]

The hierarchy from low to high in general nursing at The Cambridge Hospital and at most other hospitals in the United States, whether governmental or private, nonprofit or proprietary, is as follows:

Group A	1) Nurse's aide
	2) Orderly
Group B	3) Licensed practical nurse
	4) Registered nurse; graduate registered nurse
Group C	5) Head nurse
	6) Nurse supervisor
	7) Director of nursing

Group D   8) Intern
                 9) Resident
                 10) Chief of medicine

With few exceptions, there is no vertical mobility among Groups A, B, C, and D. Should a nurse's aide or an orderly have the desire and ability to rise to the position of LPN, previous training and experience would not be credited toward the requirements of the higher occupation. Should an LPN have the desire and ability to become a registered nurse or any of the occupations in Group C, previous training and experience are of no formal value. The LPN must start from scratch at a traditional school of nursing in order to earn a degree as a registered nurse or graduate registered nurse.[5] The principal exception in this structure is the registered nurse, who can move from Group B to Group C without a major hurdle. However, should a person in Group C have the ability and desire to become a physician, no credit is given for previous formal training and experience.

From the findings in this research project one must conclude that the lack of vertical mobility is inefficient and wasteful in terms of use of medical manpower.

The specific recommendations to The Cambridge Hospital were aimed at restructuring the functions of various occupations and increasing the opportunities for upward mobility. The principal recommendations were for —

1. an increased use of lower level personnel, such as nurse's aides and nursing assistants, to complement and to a certain extent supplant the use of RNs and LPNs on lower level, easy functions;

2. a restructuring of the jobs of RNs and LPNs, so they would perform fewer of the lower level, easy functions;

3. in-service training that would allow nurse's aides to advance to the position of nursing assistant;

4. in-service training that would allow nursing assistants to rise to the position of medical assistant;

5. in-service training that would allow medical assistants to rise to the position of physician's assistant.

In effect, the recommendations included a new occupational ladder parallel to the traditional occupational hierarchy but without the built-in historical restrictions that exist in the current structure. The new occupational ladder would permit a more efficient utilization of the talents of persons in the various occupations by eliminating arbitrary restrictions and by allowing the transfer of training and experience from one occupation to another.

As of the end of August 1971, approximately nine months after the recommendations had been made to The Cambridge Hospital, the following had occurred:

1. An in-service training program was scheduled to begin in September 1971 to upgrade nurse's aides, who are entry-level personnel, to the new occupation of nursing assistant;

2. The position of physician's assistant had been established in the medical department of the hospital, and three former Navy corpsmen were receiving in-service training for this new occupation. The Cambridge Hospital had given letters of intent to employ the physician's assistants who successfully completed the eighteen-month training program at Northeastern University;

3. In-service education programs had been instituted as recommended for the RNs and LPNs.

4. RNs were performing fewer Group I functions (easy functions) and a significant number of nurse's aides had been hired to perform these tasks;

5. Approval had been given to provide salary increases for all health personnel who successfully completed any in-service upgrading program;

6. The radiologic technicians were attending weekly conferences of surgeons to receive explanations of new procedures and techniques;

7. A number of nursing personnel (RNs and LPNs) had been exposed to previously nonexistent training in the use of EKG equipment;

8. The inhalation therapy technicians were offered occasional lectures on techniques by the department head. No formal in-service training program had yet been instituted;

9. The hiring-in requirement of a high school education for NAs was dropped;

10. Psychiatric attendants were no longer required to be high school graduates;

11. The specialized practical experience requirement for hematology specialists was reduced from two years to one.

The distribution of employment in the nursing occupations in The Cambridge Hospital changed substantially from 1969 to 1971. Over the two-year period the number of registered nurses rose by only 6.7 percent, while LPNs increased by 67.5 percent and NAs increased by 70.9 percent. If one isolated the structural changes in occupational employment, it was estimated, the wage bill for nursing personnel would have been reduced by 2.5 percent from 1969 to 1971.

The completion of this study in 1972 indicated that it was possible for a hospital to institute numerous changes that could improve the utilization of its allied health manpower. However, The Cambridge Hospital is a medium-sized municipal hospital with certain characteristics. The question remained: Can the process be repeated in numerous hospitals?

In order to determine the validity of its previous findings and to determine whether the restructuring process can be repeated in other hospitals, the Center for Medical Manpower Studies undertook a follow-up project, entitled *Improving the Utilization of Health Manpower*. Five New England hospitals with quite different characteristics were selected for the study. The five can be briefly described as follows:

Hospital A: a large short-term municipal teaching hospital (pediatrics only) serving low-income residents of the inner city.

Hospital B: a short-term private general nonprofit teaching hospital with 350 beds. It serves an upper- and middle-income urban population.

Hospital C: a large short-term private nonprofit hospital of 350 beds serving a rural population of varied incomes.

Hospital D: a short-term private nonprofit hospital of 60 beds serving a low-income urban population.

Hospital E: a 200-bed short-term general municipal teaching hospital serving a large low- and lower-middle-income urban population.

Although the data from this study are still in preliminary form, there are clear indications that the findings of the previous studies will be substantiated. Because of the inclusion of institutions with well-established in-service and upgrading programs for entry-level personnel, the comparisons of the utilization of various categories of health manpower will be considerably more pointed. Physicians, interns, residents, pediatric nurse practitioners, and nurse practitioners have been included in this study, along with the occupations previously studied. Further, this study is exploring the development of research techniques for measuring how much change in the quality of medical services has evolved through occupational restructuring and improvement in the utilization of manpower. In line with this task, there was compiled a list of "marginal medical functions" functions that generally are performed by physicians but could be performed by health personnel other than physicians.

Table 17 combines general nursing functions by degree of difficulty into three principal groups for Hospitals A, B, D, and E. Each group represents duties increasing in difficulty (Group 1, functions 1-18, the easiest; Group 3, functions 31-47, more difficult in terms of required training, on-the-job training, and professional skill).

A substantial majority of persons in each occupational group performed the easiest functions. Performing these easy functions the RNs spent 27.5 percent of their time, the LPNs 29.6 percent of their time, and the NAs 53.2 percent of their time. Group 3 functions, the more difficult nonsupervisory functions, were performed by 76.1 percent of the RNs, 77.5 percent of the LPNs, and 49.2 percent of the NAs. It is significant to note that, although the average percentage of time spent on the more difficult functions increased as the level of formal training increased, the NAs spent 12 percent of their time on these functions.

Table 18 shows the same data for Hospital C, which is engaged in extensive in-service and on-the-job training programs at all levels. A similar overlap is apparent in the performance of the easiest functions, which nearly all personnel in each occupation perform. Here, however, the RNs spend only 20.5 percent of their time on the easy functions, compared to 27.5 percent in other hospitals. LPNs perform the Group 1 tasks 31.1 percent of the time, NAs 45.7 percent of the time. RNs spent more time — 38.3 percent — in administrative and supervisory functions (miscellaneous category). Because of the effective use of on-the-job training the nurse's aides have been successfully upgraded so that they perform Group 2 functions 33.8 percent of the time and Group 3 functions 11.8 percent of the time.

Table 17. Percentage of Total Working Time Spent on Three Groups
of Functions (1), and Average Percentage Performing Within
Each Group of Functions (2), at Four New England Hospitals

Groups of Functions (ranked from easiest to most difficult)	Hospitals A, B, D, and E					
	RN		LPN		NA	
General Nursing	(1)	(2)	(1)	(2)	(1)	(2)
Group 1 (1-18)	27.5	71.3	29.6	83.7	53.2	79.4
Group 2 (19-30)	23.7	82.4	30.1	87.9	28.8	70.2
Group 3 (31-47)	26.2	76.1	19.4	77.5	12.0	49.2
Miscellaneous	22.6	—[a]	20.8	—[a]	5.9	—[a]

Source: Preliminary data, Center for Medical Manpower Studies.

[a] Not calculated for this category.

Summary

The research reviewed in this chapter clearly indicates that there is a whole range of barriers, imposed or permitted by different interest groups, that prevent the optimal utilization of health personnel. The inefficient utilization of manpower means higher costs for the users of health services and few job opportunities for the poor, the disadvantaged, and those with little education. A summary of the findings would include the following:

1. Hiring standards artificially higher than needed to perform basic tasks are common. At entry-level jobs such standards keep the disadvantaged from gaining jobs in the industry.

2. Educational requirements and institutional barriers prevent upward mobility among allied health workers, and overly rigid separation between types of workers makes even lateral mobility difficult.

3. It is difficult to acquire training for promotion or to keep up-to-date in one's occupation because of the lack of in-service or on-the-job training. Most jobs are dead-end.

4. Regardless of the difficulty of the task or the educational background of the personnel involved, there is a great deal of overlap in the performance of functions at all hospitals studied.

Table 18. Percentage of Total Working Time Spent on Three Groups
of Functions (1), and Average Percentage Performing Within
Each Group of Functions (2), at a New England Hospital

Groups of Functions (ranked from easiest to most difficult)	Hospital C					
	RN		LPN		NA	
General Nursing	(1)	(2)	(1)	(2)	(1)	(2)
Group 1 (1-18)	20.5	80.0	31.1	90.0	45.7	93.0
Group 2 (19-30)	16.0	84.0	29.7	86.6	33.8	74.2
Group 3 (31-47)	25.2	86.0	22.1	83.2	11.8	54.6
Miscellaneous	38.3	—[a]	17.0	—[a]	8.6	—[a]

Source: Preliminary data, Center for Medical Manpower Studies.

[a] Not calculated for this category.

5. Although the more difficult functions are usually performed by the more professionally trained staff members, the less-skilled allied health personnel more than occasionally perform these functions.

Research at the five hospitals indicates that changes in the utilization of health manpower can be made. Hiring standards can be lowered for many entry-level jobs. The allied health occupational hierarchy can be restructured so as to permit some upward mobility. In-service and on-the-job training can be offered to allied health personnel so as to permit wider job opportunities.

The changes that are being made and have been made in a small number of hospitals indicate that similar changes can be made in many other hospitals. But such changes are not enough for optimal utilization of allied health manpower. A major overhaul of the practices of licensing and certification must be made, and such action should be taken by the professional organizations and by various levels of government.

6

Comparisons of Health Manpower Utilization:
United States and Selected European Countries

Two trends relating to health and health manpower seem to transcend the International borders of most Western European countries and the United States. First, in most nations that belong to the Organization for Economic Cooperation and Development (OECD), the labor force employed in health care areas represents a significant and growing element of the total labor force. The health care industry usually ranks as one of the five largest fields of employment, and in most OECD countries approximately 3 to 5 percent of the labor force finds employment in this area. As shown in Table 19, from the early 1960's to the late 1960's the OECD countries had substantial increases in health manpower, in each case larger than the rise in the total labor force.

The second trend that transcends international borders seems to be the ever-increasing specialization found in all health care systems. In the United States, as reported earlier, the number of health care occupations over the last fifty years has increased from three to well over 400. Similar trends can be documented in almost all of the OECD countries. As shown in Table 20, the very substantial use of medical technicians in Italy, the Netherlands, and England; nursing assistants in Denmark, Germany, and England; and nurse-midwives in all countries attest to the increasing complexity and fragmentation of medical services.

Between 1900 and 1950 modern medicine in the United States had an enormous positive impact on the effects of disease: alleviating suffering, terminating severe illness, preventing crippling, and postponing untimely death. These changes have been closely associated with increased standards of living, better housing, and improved educational opportunities. Drugs like penicillin provide immediate cure of diseases such as lobar pneumonia, which decades ago claimed one-quarter of its victims.

As a result of these changes from 1900 to 1950 there has been a decrease in infant mortality and a general increase in life expectancy. But despite the enormous expansion of medical facilities, expenditures on medical research, and increases in health manpower in the subsequent twenty-five years, there has been a steady leveling-off in our health progress. Dr. David Rutstein of the Harvard Medical School described this enormous expansion of medical research, facilities, and manpower together with our lagging national health picture as the paradox of modern medicine in the United States.[1]

Between 1965 and 1972 expenditures on health care in the United States skyrocketed from $39 billion to $89.5 billion, representing an increase from 5.9 percent to 7.7 percent of the gross national product (GNP). Per capita expenditures on health care in 1972 amounted to $422, up $43 (11.4 percent). In 1972 third-party payers met 90 percent of the hospital bill, 58 percent of the physician's bill, 13 percent of the bill for dental care and drugs, and 60 percent of the total spent for other services. Despite these changes, there was an 8.5 percent increase in direct per capita payments over the 1971 figure.[2]

These increases in expenditures and costs notwithstanding, the United States has failed to improve the health status of its population substantially over the past decade. The major health indices — average life expectancy at birth and infant mortality — show very little improvement in recent years.

Although major health problems still vary from one country to another, the general health status has improved in most European nations over the past twenty years. Comparisons of some of the

Table 19. Percentage of Total Labor Force Engaged in the Health Care Industry in Selected OECD Countries, Selected Years 1960-1970

	Year	Total Labor Force	Health Care Personnel Number of Persons	Health Care Personnel Percentage of Total Labor Force
Australia	1961	4,225,096	134,453	3.2
	1966	4,856,455	190,672	3.9
Canada	1961	6,471,850	307,515	4.8
	1970	8,374,000	502,282	6.0
Denmark	1960	2,007,639	76,981	3.8
	1965	2,198,628	94,407	4.3
France	1962	18,956,380	536,160	2.8
	1968	20,002,240	730,660	3.7
Greece	1961	3,638,601	38,708	1.1
	1971	3,283,880	40,680	1.2
Ireland (Republic of)	1961	1,052,539	30,331	2.9
	1966	1,065,987	33,576	3.1
Japan	1960	43,690,500	647,266	1.5
	1971	50,630,000	961,000	1.9
New Zealand	1961	895,363	37,237	4.2
	1966	1,026,039	44,608	4.3
Sweden	1960	3,244,084	119,391	3.7
	1970	3,412,668	210,407	6.2
United Kingdom	1960	25,072,000	774,000	3.1
	1970	25,675,000	1,037,000	4.0
United States	1960	72,142,000	2,642,300	3.7
	1970	85,903,000	4,246,187	4.9

Source: Centre for Educational Research and Development, *New Directions in Education for Changing Health Care Systems* (Paris: Organization for Economic Cooperation and Development, 1975), p. 32.

Table 20. Number of Persons Engaged in Various Health Occupations in Selected Industrialized Countries

Country	Physicians		Midwives	Nurses	Nursing Assistants	Physiotherapists	Technicians
	Number	Population Per Physician					
Belgium	15,500	630	3,333	n.a.	n.a.	n.a.	n.a.
Denmark	7,000	700	580	26,000[a]	11,620[b]	2,340	n.a.
France	71,000	721	9,000	150,000	150,000	20,500	n.a.
West Germany	114,771	572	6,505	185,792	2,748	19,856	15,934[c]
Ireland	3,011	960	d	16,067	n.a.	n.a.	n.a.
Italy[e]	99,341	544[f]	18,828	127,399	g	n.a.	156,055[g]
Luxembourg	368	924	90	667[h]	h	n.a.	n.a.
Netherlands	17,381	760	883	50,114[j]	n.a.	1,195	6,971[k]
England and Wales	70,122	771	19,258	180,679	99,927	7,687	7,045
United States[l]	322,000	641	4,950	1,175,000[m]	875,000	15,000	145,000[n]

Source: Unless otherwise stipulated, sources for all data are from World Health Organization, *Health Services in Europe* (Copenhagen: 1975). Additional sources and verification are from United Nations, *Demographic Yearbook 1972* (New York: 1973), *World Health Statistics Report 26* (Copenhagen: 1973). Most figures are for 1970, although some are for 1969 and 1971.

n.a. – either not available or occupation does not exist.

a One-third are part-time.

b One-quarter are part-time..

cSurgery and laboratory assistants.

d Listed with nurses.

e Data for Italy are from *United Nations, Statistical Yearbook, 1974*, p. 784.

f Includes dentists. Dentists must first earn an M.D. before specializing in dentistry.

g Includes nursing aides, laboratory assistants, and radiologic technicians, from *Annuario Di Statistiche Sanitarie, 1971-72*

h Nurses and nursing assistants are totaled together.

jIncludes public health nurses and student nurses.

k Includes radiologic and laboratory technicians.

l Data for the United States are from *Health Resources Statistics, 1972-73*, pp. 8-11.

mIncludes RNs and LPNs.

nLaboratory technologists and technicians.

most industrial nations of Europe with the United States demonstrate that most have made significant progress in improving the quality of health care while the United States has not made much headway. There has been a continuous decline in infant mortality rates accompanied by a lengthening average life expectancy at birth. The age distribution of the population in these nations has shifted so that the over-60 age group accounts for more than 15 percent — and in some cases, 20 percent — of the population.[3]

However, the most outstanding improvement in health status has been in the younger age groups. The median infant mortality rate in European nations decreased from 30 to about 20 per 1,000 live births between 1962 and 1972.[4] In great measure these substantial decreases in infant mortality rates are due directly to the significant increase in the number of allied health personnel.

In some of these countries one of the more obvious factors in the utilization of health manpower is the employment of nurse-midwives. Although there were almost 5,000 nurse-midwives in the United States in 1972, their activity and impact was only marginal because of the relatively small number and the legal limitations placed on them by most states. In the Western European countries that rely heavily on nurse-midwives, there is a strong correlation between the established system of prenatal and delivery care and the low infant mortality rates. It has been shown that the probabilities of complications for both the mother and child are significantly decreased if the mother receives proper care from early in the pregnancy. In the United States the health system fails to provide equal access to such early care for all levels of society, and this failure results in an unacceptable level of infant mortality among nonwhites (29 per 1,000 in 1972). The use of nurse-midwives, a health occupation for which one could readily be trained on the job, is strongly correlated with low infant mortality rates.

Were the quality of health care assured by the ratio of physicians to total population, Italy, for example, would easily outrank the United States. In December 1974 Italy had approximately 114,000 active physicians, yielding a ratio of one physician for every 518 members of the population. In the United States, the ratio was one physician for 733 members of the population.

Because of the maldistribution of physicians and the general lack of ambulatory facilities, the Italian health delivery system is heavily dependent on its in-hospital nursing personnel. However, there is a severe shortage of trained registered nurses, and in 1974 Italy had only eight active registered nurses per 10,000 population; in the United States the figure was 35.3 per 10,000 population. The World Health Organization has set an optimum figure of 30 per 10,000 population. Unlike in the United States, outpatient facilities in Italy are practically nonexistent, and in 1971 it had less than 10,000 allied health employees functioning outside of traditional in-patient hospital facilities. The ratio of allied health personnel working outside the hospital inpatient environment was one per 3,562 persons in Italy and one per 129 persons in the United States. If manpower is a key factor in furnishing a sufficient quantity and a high quality of health services, it would appear that the availability of qualified allied health personnel is more important than the availability of physicians.

7

The Future of Allied Health Manpower

The future of allied health manpower and the roles these workers will play are dependent on the health care priorities set at the national level of our government but are modified to some extent by the pressures exerted by the public at large. In the pursuit of health Americans can travel several different roads. The avenues of change selected will have a direct impact on the quantity and varieties of allied health manpower employed by the health industry over the next several decades.

If, for example, one of the nation's health goals becomes the complete eradication in the near future of the major fatal diseases of stroke, cancer, and heart disease, it would mean a tremendous increase in the demand for a particular mix of health manpower, with varying degrees of professional and in-service training. If such a program were successful, according to some calculations, average life expectancy at birth would be extended by only approximately six or seven years. And at age 65, average life expectancy would be extended by no more than one-and-a-half or two years.[1] Alternately, if the nation's aim is to have the most positive impact on healthiness and longevity, Dr. Lester Breslow and his staff at the School of Public Health of the University of California-Los Angeles would point our efforts in a different direction. Dr. Breslow investigated the impact of various health practices on health status; seven independent guidelines with strong correlations to longevity and healthiness were discovered. These guidelines are — (1) do not smoke cigarettes, (2) sleep seven hours each day, (3) eat breakfast, (4) keep your weight down, (5) drink moderately, (6) exercise daily, and (7) do not eat between meals. As noted by Dr. Kass, a regular check-up visit to a physician is conspicuous by its absence. This study noted that the health status of persons over 75 years of age who conscientiously pursued all seven guidelines was very similar to the general health status of persons aged 35 to 44 who pursued fewer than three guidelines. Further, the study indicated that persons pursuing at least six of the seven guidelines had a life expectancy eleven years longer at age 45 than persons who followed less than four. Finally, the variances in health status directly associated with the seven guidelines were evident at all economic levels and, except at income levels below subsistence, appeared to be largely independent of income.[2] Such a health goal would require a radically different mix of health personnel, with a much greater potential for the employment of persons with less formal schooling.

We have mentioned two diametrically opposite options, but any combination of the above with other alternatives is possible. Each option or goal would require a different size and mix of health manpower. In the field of medical care, change in the delivery system is probably the name of the game over the next decade. Dr. David Rutstein put it this way:

Actually, if medical care remains in its present chaotic state, there simply will never be enough physicians, nurses, or other medical personnel to do the job. Physicians will continue to be overconcentrated in suburban areas and will be impossible to find in the jungles of our large cities and in our wide open rural spaces. General physician services will become even more scarce.[3]

The Implications of a National Health Insurance Program

National health insurance in the United States has had a fairly long but unresolved history — from commission reports in 1910, support from the American Federation of Labor in the mid-1930's, support from President Harry S. Truman in 1949, and the introduction of sixteen different bills in the United States 93rd Congress. Private health insurance plans partly protect almost 90 percent of the civilian population under age 65, principally against emergency and catastrophic occurrences, and pay for approximately two-fifths of the health care costs of those covered. Private insurance companies and Blue Cross-Blue Shield also offer extensive plan coverage, but the higher costs are sufficient to discourage many from increasing their protection. Some, though not the majority, of the current proposals for national health insurance do concern themselves with and provide assistance for health manpower shortages and maldistribution problems that would result from the adoption of the proposed plan.

The basic provisions of the national health insurance proposals now before Congress fall into two broad categories: full-coverage plans and coinsurance or deductible plans.[4] The former provides for full coverage of all services. Coinsurance requires out-of-pocket payment of some fixed percentage of each dollar spent for health services. A deductible provision requires that all initial costs up to a specified amount be paid before the insurance becomes effective. The researchers Newhouse, Phelps, and Schwartz examine how these two basic types of plans affect inpatient services and ambulatory services.

Inpatient Services

Because most inpatient services are currently covered by either private or government insurance programs, the increase in demand for such services resulting from any form of national health insurance would be relatively small. However, since inpatient services constitute more than half of the $62 billion spent annually on health services, a small relative change in demand would result in a large absolute shift in resources devoted to health care. If 90 percent of all inpatient bills were paid by third parties, a full-coverage plan would expand protection by 10 percent, which could lead to an increase of about 5 to 15 percent in demand for inpatient services. The effect of a 25-percent maximum coinsurance plan would be less and could range from nothing to 8 percent.

Ambulatory Services

Unlike inpatient hospital care, expanded coverage of ambulatory services would result in a large percentage increase in demand. For ambulatory physician services Newhouse, Phelps, and Schwartz estimated that a full-coverage plan would increase demand by 75 percent, and that a 25-percent maximum coinsurance plan would increase demand by 30 percent. The authors noted that these represent conservative estimates of the changes that can be expected under each program. And for related allied health services they concluded that a full-coverage plan would increase demand for allied health services by 35 to 40 percent, a 25-percent coinsurance plan by approximately 15 percent.

The authors of that study readily admit that their estimates are conservative. To obtain reliable estimates one would first have to make a prediction as to the specific form and substance of the health insurance plan that will become law. From the terms of this law one would then have to apply sophisticated forecasting techniques in order to get more reliable estimates of the effects on the demand for health services. And a final step in the procedure would be to convert the increase in the demand for health services into changes in the demand for allied health personnel. The experts have not yet reached this point of forecasting the specific effects of a national health insurance law.

An educated guess could put the overall effects on the employment of allied health manpower of a likely national health insurance law at about 50 percent. Assuming such a plan could be implemented in about four years, the growth rate of health personnel would have to exceed 10 percent merely to cover the needs of the plan's new coverage. But there are many other factors that are increasing the demand for health personnel, and the annual growth rate is likely to be closer to 20 percent than to 10 percent. Job opportunities at all levels of the occupational hierarchy will be substantial. The proportion of these job opportunities at the entry level that will be open to the disadvantaged and not dead-end will depend on the changes which the industry is prepared to make. This report has shown that changes can be made in the industry.

The Implications of an Affluent Society

As the American society has become more affluent over the past thirty years, greater emphasis has been placed on education. A growing proportion of the population has completed high school, and a rising percentage of high school completers are entering and graduating from two-year and four-year institutions of higher learning. The American society is spending a growing proportion of its income on personal services, including education and health. And as a larger proportion of the American people receive some higher education, their demand for health services has increased. But more than just an increase in the demand for health services, there has been a significant change over the past few years in attitudes toward the health care industry.

The increase in the demand for health service has meant a need not only for more physicians, but also for more health facilities and for the necessary allied health personnel to service the facilities. And if this trend of seeking "more health" continues, the demand for physicians will far outstrip the supply, and only by a substitution of allied health personnel for physicians will the demand for health services in the future possibly be met.

In the past the professional opinions of physicians were accepted without question. The medical doctor was traditionally looked upon as a source of knowledge and wisdom. Recently, however, the professional status of physicians has been battered, as more of the public question the capability of physicians to handle the problems of sickness and disease. Consumers of health care services are asking physicians more penetrating questions and demanding technical medical answers. They are seeking the consultative services of a variety of specialists. They are refusing to accept errors in judgment with tranquility or finality, and they are filing a growing number of malpractice suits in the courts. Professional monitoring groups are assuming greater responsibilities; and certificate of need committees, peer review groups, specialty boards, and tissue committees are becoming increasingly involved in the medical care process.

This entire trend is leading and will continue to lead to a more cautious practice of medicine by all, now called the practice of defensive medicine: consultations will be more common, laboratory testing will be utilized more frequently, and radiology will experience a substantial growth, along with pharmacy, nursing, and every level of health care. The burgeoning effects of this trend will undoubtedly mean a continued growth in the demand for allied health personnel.

The affluence of our society may partly explain the increased efforts in scientific and technological research and discoveries in the health area, as well as increases in concern over maximum health care. These changes had significant impact on the utilization of allied health manpower. Between 1950 and 1970, for example, the number of allied health workers rose from approximately 1.2 million to 3.9 million, while the number of physicians to other types of health workers dropped from a ratio of 15 to 100 to a ratio of 8 to 100. According to one study,[5] part of this demand was the result of expanding biomedical research, part was due to new technologies, and part arose from new concepts of maximum health care. And this growth in allied health manpower took two forms: (1) increased numbers of traditional workers, such as nurse's aides, registered nurses, and laboratory technicians; and (2) the introduction of new occupational titles, such as electroencephalographic technician, physician's assistant, and biostatistician.

As more funds and effort are put into scientific research to discover cures or solutions to our many health problems, the demand for health workers will increase.

Allied Health Personnel vs. the Physician

A substantial part of the growth in the number of allied health occupations has been at the expense of functions at one time performed by physicians. As the demand for physicians' services expanded faster than the supply of practicing physicians, the rate of encroachment by allied health personnel on the functions of physicians increased. In recent years there has been an acceleration of the process as the increase in the number of practicing physicians failed to keep pace with the population growth. New occupations, such as medic and physician's assistant, have been recently developed, in which specific physician functions are assigned and are generally performed under the direct supervision of the physician. Other such health occupations are sure to be developed in the future.

In a study currently in progress a comparison is made of the medical functions usually performed by various categories of health manpower, the frequency of the performance, and the level of medical sophistication of the function.[6] In one comparison, sixty-nine nursing functions, which encompass 100 percent of nursing time, were ranked in order of difficulty and then tested against the actual performance of registered nurses, licensed practical nurses, nurse's aides, and physicians. A preliminary examination of the data indicates that the physicians perform virtually all of the sixty-nine functions, and that approximately 40 percent of the physicians' time is spent performing these functions.

In a second comparison 279 functions, including the sixty-nine nursing functions plus those traditionally performed by the physician, were ranked in order of difficulty and then tested against the performance of physicians, registered nurses, nurse practitioners, and pediatric nurse practitioners. Interestingly, all four occupations performed very similar medical functions for a majority of time spent on the job. The physicians were found to be performing and spending significant amounts of time on the medical functions performed by the other health manpower personnel who had received considerably less sophisticated formal training. The reverse also holds. The less-trained personnel performed many of the functions traditionally performed by the physicians. Physicians themselves are often quoted as saying they spend three-quarters of their time on medical functions that have been adequately performed by other levels of health manpower.

If the projected growth rate in the demand for health services materializes, the relative shortage of practicing physicians will grow substantially. There is little possibility that the supply of physicians can keep pace with the demand. The result of such growing shortage is likely to be a general upgrading of occupations in the medical occupational ladder. Nursing occupations will quickly assume a growing proportion of the functions physicians would perform, if there were sufficient physicians. As this happens, greater opportunities for upward mobility will be available for persons in the entry-level positions.

Job Opportunities in the Future

In the last decade there has been substantial growth in the health care industry in the United States and throughout the world. Since the industry is very labor-intensive, the growth has meant a significant increase in the number of persons employed. A rather large proportion of the industry's employment could be classified as unskilled or semiskilled, which theoretically could have meant many job opportunities for the disadvantaged. However, because of arbitrary hiring standards, especially those related to education and training, many of the disadvantaged were excluded from the industry. Because of institutional barriers and rigid descriptions of occupations and job requirements (including licensing and certification), many of the disadvantaged who managed to get into the industry found themselves in monotonous, dead-end jobs, with no real opportunity for advancement. Wages of allied health manpower have improved considerably over the past ten years, but on the average their earnings still are approximately 10 percent below those of workers of similar education, training, and skill level in the industrial sector.

It would appear that the disadvantaged job seekers — the black, the Spanish-speaking, the high-school dropout — have not gotten their fair share of the better job opportunities in the rapidly growing health care industry. Gains have been made, but there are many more still to be made.

What of the future of this industry and of the industry's job opportunities for the disadvantaged, whose unemployment rates in some categories are double that of the national average? Can we afford to be optimistic?

For the industry as a whole, the future looks very rosy. There is little doubt that over the next decade there will be a substantial growth in the industry, and therefore in the employment of health personnel. There are many factors that lead to this conclusion —

1. the current growth rate of inpatient facilities

2. the current development and growth of ambulatory facilities

3. the current growth rate of extended care facilities

4. the upward trend in the sophistication level of medical care and service

5. the growing level of expectation of health services by American consumers

6. the gradual but continuing encroachment of allied health personnel on the functions traditionally performed by physicians

7. the normal growth in demand for health services due to population growth

8. the probable passage of a national health insurance program.

In 1973 there were close to 6 million persons whose longest work experience during that year was in the medical and health services industry.[7] It has been estimated that average employment in the industry is about 4.5 million, with a substantial majority employed in hospitals. Of that 4.5 million persons in the health care industry almost 45 percent can be considered to be employed in entry-level or near entry-level occupations.

As indicated above, our estimate of the effects a national health insurance program would have on the demand for manpower is about a 50 percent rise. The normal growth of the population, plus all the other factors that increase the demand for health services are likely to mean an additional increase of at least 10 percent per year in the demand for allied health employees. In this very substantial increase in health service demand there is a built-in factor that leads to a more-than-proportionate rise in the demand for workers in the lower-level occupations. Because of the lead time needed to increase the supply of physicians and other health professionals requiring some college or university training, and because of the institutional barriers limiting the supply of such high-level professionals, any significant increase in the demand for health services will result in a substitution of employees with low-level skills for employees at the higher-level occupations. Will the health providers recognize the opportunity they have of offering meaningful job opportunities to the disadvantaged?

The problem is how to short-circuit the cumbersome and irrational but traditional employment barriers in medical centers that prevent or impede entry-level personnel from reaching their full potential within some realistic occupational structure. We have documented in this report that some medical institutions have overcome this difficult barrier. The University of Chicago Hospitals, the Eastern Maine Medical Center, and The Cambridge Hospital have made significant strides in this area. Other institutions have been successful in reordering their occupational priorities in an attempt to overcome useless but traditional occupational barriers. Still others are currently studying the problem, with the intention of trying to make changes in the near future. We are convinced that the restructuring of allied health occupations along more rational lines can be accomplished by a majority of health providers across the nation. If the restructuring of health occupations can be successful in dozens of medical institutions, only the lack of strong motivation and interest prevents success by other health providers.

A rational restructuring of the occupational hierarchy of a hospital will result in a more meaningful and satisfying work experience for the allied health worker. Medical costs are not likely to decline as a result of such changes. However, there is a reasonable possibility that the development of realistic, restructured health occupations, with attainable job satisfaction, would dampen the trend of rapidly rising medical costs. A satisfied worker is more productive, and having more satisfied workers results in lower labor turnover.

The health of the nation can certainly be improved. Job opportunities in the health industry will certainly increase. Will the disadvantaged get their fair share of meaningful jobs in the industry? If serious efforts are made to change the structure and eliminate barriers, we will succeed.

Notes

CHAPTER 1

1. Sar A. Levitan, *Programs in Aid of the Poor for the 1970's,* rev. ed. (Baltimore: The Johns Hopkins University Press, Policy Studies in Employment and Welfare, 1973). p.7.

2. National Center for Health Statistics, *Health Resources Statistics, 1974* (Rockville, Md.; U.S. Department of Health, Education and Welfare, Health Resources Administration, Public Health Service, 1974), pp. 517-533.

3. Unpublished estimates from National Center for Health Statistics, January 1976.

4. Victor R. Fuchs, *Who Shall Live? Health, Economics, and Social Choice* (New York: Basic Books, 1974), pp. 3-29. Also see Leon R. Kass, "Regarding the End of Medicine and the Pursuit of Health," *The Public Interest* no. 40 (Summer 1975), pp. 11-42.

5. Milton I. Roemer and Jay W. Friedman, *Doctors in Hospitals* (Baltimore: The Johns Hopkins University Press, 1971), p. 34.

6. Abraham Flexner, *The Flexner Report on Medical Education in the United States and Canada* (Washington: The Carnegie Foundation, Science and Health Publications, 1910); reprinted 1960.

7. American Hospital Association, *Hospital Statistics,* Annual Survey, 1974 edition (Chicago: AHA, 1974), p. 7.

8. *Ibid.*

9. William J. Bicknell and Diana Chapman Walsh, "Certification-of-Need: The Massachusetts Experience," *New England Journal of Medicine* vol. 292, no. 20 (May 15, 1975), pp. 1054-1061.

CHAPTER 2

1. Dean S. Ammer, *Institutional Employment and Shortage of Paramedical Personnel: A Detailed Study of Staffing in Hospitals, Nursing Homes, and Various Institutions in the Greater Boston Area,* under a grant from the U.S. Public Health Service (Boston: Northeastern University Press, 1967), p. v.

2. Eli Ginzberg and Miriam Ostow, *Men, Money, and Medicine* (New York: Columbia University Press, 1969), pp. 133-134.

3. Committee for Economic Development, *Building a National Health Care System* (New York: CED, 1973), p. 33.

4. Bureau of Labor Statistics, *Annual Earnings and Employment Patterns of Private Non-Agricultural Employees, 1965* (Washington: U.S. Department of Labor, 1970), Bulletin 1675, Table 1, pp. 9-10. Also see Bureau of Labor Statistics, *Industry Wage Survey, Hospitals, March 1969* (Washington: U.S. Department of Labor, 1971), Bulletin 1688, pp. 14-15. These data include all hospitals except those operated by the federal government.

5. Harry I. Greenfield (with the assistance of Carol A. Brown), *Allied Health Manpower: Trends and Prospects* (New York: Columbia University Press, 1969), p. vii.

6. Ginzberg and Ostow, *Men, Money, and Medicine,* p. 153.

7. Morris A. Horowitz and Harold M. Goldstein, *Hiring Standards for Paramedical Manpower,* under a grant from the U.S. Department of Labor, Manpower Administration (Boston: Northeastern University, 1968). Available from the National Technical Information Service (NTIS), Springfield, Va. 22152, accession no. PB-179846.

8. Three years was chosen somewhat arbitrarily as a period long enough for the worker both to display an attachment to the job and to make a fairly realistic assessment of the chances for advancement.

9. Goldstein and Horowitz, *Restructuring Paramedical Occupations: A Case Study,* Final Report, under a contract with the U.S. Department of Labor, Manpower Administration, 2 vols. (Boston: Northeastern University, 1972). Available from NTIS, accession nos. PB-211113 (vol. 1), PB-211114 (vol. 2; Appendix C, Definition of Tasks and Functions; Appendix D, Phase II Tables, Analyzing the Functions Performed by Paramedical Personnel).

CHAPTER 3

1. Sponsored by the Office of Research and Development, Manpower Administration, U.S. Department of Labor, this research is being done by the authors through the Center for Medical Manpower Studies, Northeastern University, Boston.

2. Massachusetts Rate Setting Commission, "Nursing Homes Statistics Questionnaire," unpublished data, 1973.

3. Horowitz and Goldstein, *Hiring Standards for Paramedical Manpower.*

4. *Ibid.*

CHAPTER 4

1. Greenfield and Brown, *Allied Health Manpower*, p. 100.

2. Martha D. Ballenger and E. Harvey Estes, Jr., "Licensure or Responsible Delegation," *New England Journal of Medicine* vol. 284, no. 6 (February 11, 1971), pp. 330-331.

3. E. H. Forgotson and Ruth Roemer, "Government Licensure and Voluntary Standards for Health Personnel and Facilities: Their Power and Limitations in Assuring High-Quality Health Care," *Medical Care* vol. 6, no. 5 (September-October 1968), p. 346.

4. National Center for Health Statistics, *Health Resources Statistics 1974*, p. 535.

5. Goldstein and Horowitz, *Restructuring Paramedical Occupations*.

6. Florence S. Stern *et al.*, "Upgrading Nurses Aides to LPNs through a Work-Study Program," Final Progress Report (New York: Medical Health Research Association of New York, 1970).

7. *Ibid.*, p. 28.

8. Sally Holloway and Robert G. Holloway, "The Development of a Program of Career Mobility in Hospitals," paper presented at the American Hospital Association Convention, Chicago, August 1971), pp. 10-25.

9. *Ibid.*, pp. 10-16.

10. Nathan Hershey, "New Directions in Licensure of Health Personnel," *Economic and Business Bulletin* vol. 24, no. 1 (Fall 1971), p. 32.

11. Nathan Hershey and Walter S. Wheeler, "Health Personnel Regulation in the Public Interest: QA on Institutional Licensure," (Sacramento: California Hospital Association 1973), pp. 13-15.

12. Randolph Tucker and Burtchaell G. Wetterau, *Credentialing Health Personnel by Licensed Hospitals: The Report of a Study of Institutional Licensure* 2 vols. (Chicago: Rush-Presbyterian-St. Luke's Medical Center, February 1975), I:11.

13. *Ibid.*, pp. 17-18.

14. *Ibid.*, p. 53.

CHAPTER 5

1. Greenfield and Brown, *Allied Health Manpower*, p. 182.

2. Goldstein and Horowitz, *Restructuring Paramedical Occupations*.

3. Before this project received assurance of federal funding, a hospital had to be found to cooperate in the project. This was a difficult task. We were refused entry by several hospitals on the grounds that the project "would be disruptive," "would create tension among various factions within the hospitals," or "would bring undesirables into the area."

4. Social Development Corporation, *Technical Assistance to Comprehensive Health Services Projects on Manpower Development* Final Progress Report, Phase I (New York: SDC, 1970), pp. 7-8.

5. There are several programs in the United States that do give advanced credit to LPNs who wish to become RNs. One such program has recently been started at Northeastern University, Boston; however, the program is limited to fifteen students. In general, such programs are full-time and require the participants to give up their jobs.

CHAPTER 6

1. David D. Rutstein, *The Coming Revolution in Medicine* (Cambridge, Mass.: MIT Press, 1967), pp. 9-48.
2. Social Security Administration, *Calendar 1972 Highlights,* pub. no. 11701 (Washington: U.S. Department of Health, Education and Welfare, 1974), p. 3.
3. *Ibid.*, p. 4.
4. *Ibid.,* p. 5.

CHAPTER 7

1. Leon R. Kass, "Regarding the End of Medicine and the Pursuit of Health," *The Public Interest,* No. 40 (Summer 1975), p. 17.
2. Nedra B. Belloc and Lester Breslow, "Relationship of Physical Health Status and Health Practices," *Preventive Medicine* 1972, pp. 409-421; and Nedra B. Belloc, "Relationship of Health Practices and Mortality," *Preventive Medicine* 1973, pp. 67-81.
3. David D. Rutstein, *Blueprint for Medical Care* (Cambridge, Mass.: MIT Press, 1974), p. 57.
4. For a detailed discussion of the possible effects of alternate insurance plans on the demand for service and manpower, see Joseph P. Newhouse, Charles E. Phelps, and William B. Schwartz, "Policy Options and the Impact of National Health Insurance," *New England Journal of Medicine* vol. 290, no. 24 (June 13, 1974), pp. 1345-1359.
5. A. M. Yohalem and C. M. Brecher, "The University Medical Center and the Metropolis: A Working Paper," in Eli Ginzberg and Alice M. Yohalem, eds., *The University Medical Center and the Metropolis* (New York: Josiah Macy, Jr., Foundation, 1974), p. 8.
6. Goldstein and Horowitz, "A Five-Hospital Study," funded by the Employment and Training Administration, U.S. Department of Labor. In process.
7. Bureau of Labor Statistics, *Handbook of Labor Statistics, 1975,* reference edition (Washington: U.S. Department of Labor, 1975), p. 101.

Selected Bibliography

American Hospital Association. *Hospital Statistics*, Annual Survey, 1974 Edition. Chicago: AHA, 1974

Ammer, Dean S. *Institutional Employment and Shortage of Paramedical Personnel: A Detailed Study of Staffing in Hospitals, Nursing Homes, and Various Institutions in the Greater Boston Area,* under a grant from the United States Public Health Service. Boston: Northeastern University Press, 1967.

Ballenger, Martha D., and Estes, E. Harvey, Jr. "Licensure or Responsible Delegation," *New England Journal of Medicine* Vol. 284, no. 6 (February 11, 1971).

Committee for Economic Development. *Building a National Health Care System.* New York: Committee for Educational Development, April 1973.

Flexner, Abraham. *The Flexner Report on Medical Education in the United States and Canada.* Washington: The Carnegie Foundation, Science and Health Publications, 1910. Reprinted 1960.

Forgotson, E.D., and Roemer, Ruth. "Government Licensure and Voluntary Standards for Health Personnel and Facilities: Their Power and Limitations in Assuring High-Quality Health Care," *Medical Care* Volume 6, no. 5 (September-October 1968).

Fuchs, Victor R. *Who Shall Live? Health Economics and Social Choice.* New York: Basic Books, 1974.

Ginzberg, Eli, and Ostow, Miriam. *Men, Money and Medicine.* New York: Columbia University Press, 1969.

Ginzberg, Eli, and Yohalem, Alice M., eds. *The University Medical Center and the Metropolis,* New York: Josiah Macy, Jr., Foundation, 1974.

Goldstein, Harold M.; Guzzanti, E.; Lancia, E.; and Schachter, Gus-
tav. "Experience of Health Care Coverage in Italy and the Impli-
cations for the United States." Proceedings of a symposium "The
New Public Service Employment and the Health Delivery System:
Research Issues and Potentialities." Washington: Bureau of
Health Services Research, National Institutes of Health, June,
1975.
Goldstein, Harold M., and Horowitz, Morris A. *Guide to Restructur-
ing Medical Manpower Occupations in Hospitals.* Boston: Spauld-
ing, 1975.
_____ *Research and Development in the Utilization of Medical
Manpower.* Boston: Spaulding, 1974.
_____ *Restructuring Paramedical Occupations.* A report to the
Manpower Administration, U.S. Department of Labor, 2 vols.
Boston: Northeastern University, 1972.
Greenfield, Harry I. (with the assistance of Carol A. Brown). *Allied
Health Manpower: Trends and Prospects.* New York: Columbia
University Press, 1969.
Hershey, Nathan. "New Directions in Licensure of Health Person-
nel," *Economic and Business Bulletin,* Vol. 24, No. 1 (Fall 1971).
Holloway, Sally, and Holloway, Robert G. "The Development of a
Program of Career Mobility in Hospitals." Paper presented at the
American Hospital Association Convention. Chicago: AHA, Aug-
ust 1971.
Horowitz, Morris A., and Goldstein, Harold M. *Hiring Standards for
Paramedical Manpower.* A report to the Manpower Administra-
tion, U.S. Department of Labor. Boston: Northeastern Univer-
sity, 1968.
Levitan, Sar A. *Programs in Aid of the Poor for the 1970's.* rev. ed.
Baltimore: The Johns Hopkins University Press, Policy Studies in
Employment and Welfare, 1973.
McCleery, Robert. *One Life — One Physician.* Washington: Public
Affairs Press, 1971.
National Center for Health Statistics. *Health Resources Statistics,
1974.* Rockville, Md.: U.S. Department of Health, Education and
Welfare, Health Resources Administration, Public Health Service,
1974.
Reinhardt, Uwe E. *Physician Productivity and the Demand for
Health Manpower.* Cambridge, Mass.: Ballinger Publishing, 1975.
Roemer, Milton I., and Friedman, Jay W. *Doctors in Hospitals.* Bal-
timore: The Johns Hopkins University Press, 1971.
Rutstein, David D. *Blueprint for Medical Care.* Cambridge, Mass.:
MIT Press, 1974.
_____ *The Coming Revolution in Medicine.* Cambridge, Mass.:
MIT Press, 1967.

Tucker, W. Randolph, and Wetterau, Burchaell G. *Credentialing Health Personnel by Licensed Hospitals: the Report of a Study of Institutional Licensure.* 2 vols. Chicago: Rush-Presbyterian-St. Luke's Medical Center, February 1975.

World Health Organization, Regional Office for Europe. *Health Service in Europe.* 2nd ed. Copenhagen: WHO, 1975.

Index

A

Admissions to hospitals, 10, 11, 12
AFL-CIO, national health insurance, 81; upgrading project, 45, 47
Affluence, effects on the demand for health services, 9, 83, 84
Allied health personnel, 5, 18, 22, 69, 79, 85; with credentials, 54-55; organizations, 17
Ambulatory, 24, 25, 77; facilities, 87; employment, 24, 26
American Hospital Association, 11, 12, 15, 89, 91, 93
Ammer, Dean, 17, 90, 93
Average daily census, 10-12
Average life expectancy, 72

B

Ballenger, Martha D., and Estes, E. Harvey, Jr., 41, 91, 93
Belloc, Nelda, 92; and Breslow, Lester, 92
Bicknell, William J., and Walsh, Diana Chapman, 89
Blue Cross-Blue Shield, 81

Boston-Cambridge Survey, 21, 24-28; employment data, 26
Breslow, Lester, 79

C

Career Mobility Program, 49
Center for Medical Manpower Studies, 26, 27, 48, 68, 69
Certificate of Need Committee (CON), 13-15
Certification (see also Licensure), 2, 6, 28, 41, 39-55, 69
Chicago Clinics and Hospital, 47
Committee for Economic Development (CED), 18, 90, 93
Community hospitals, 10
Consumer Price Index (CPI), 13

D

Defensive Medicine, 84
Demand for health services, 7, 25, 81, 83
Demand for health workers, 17, 19, 21, 84
Demand for physician's services, 20,

Library of Congress Cataloging in Publication Data

Goldstein, Harold M   1930-
    Entry-level health occupations.

    (Policy studies in employment and welfare: no. 27)
    Bibliography: p. 93
    1. Allied health personnel – Employment – United States. I. Horowitz, Morris Aaron, joint author. II. Title. [DNLM: 1. Allied health personnel – Utilization. W21.5 G624u]
RA410.7.G64   610.69′53′0973   76-41270
ISBN 0-8018-1911-3
ISBN 0-8018-1912-1 pbk.